Revisiting Waterbirth

WITHDRAWN

Revisiting Waterbirth

An Attitude to Care

Dianne Garland

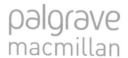

First published 2011 by
PALGRAVE MACMILLAN

Palgrave Macmillan in the UK is an imprint of Macmillan Publishers Limited, registered in England, company number 785998, of Houndmills, Basingstoke, Hampshire RG21 6XS.

Palgrave Macmillan in the US is a division of St Martin's Press LLC, 175 Fifth Avenue, New York, NY 10010.

Palgrave Macmillan is the global academic imprint of the above companies and has companies and representatives throughout the world.

Palgrave® and Macmillan® are registered trademarks in the United States, the United Kingdom, Europe and other countries

ISBN 978–0–230–27357–3

This book is based upon *Waterbirth*, the author's previous book, and includes some material from it. First edition published 1995 by Butterworth Heinemann Ltd. Second edition published 2000 by Books for Midwives.

This book is printed on paper suitable for recycling and made from fully managed and sustained forest sources. Logging, pulping and manufacturing processes are expected to conform to the environmental regulations of the country of origin.

A catalogue record for this book is available from the British Library.

A catalog record for this book is available from the Library of Congress.

10   9   8   7   6   5   4   3   2   1
20   19   18   17   16   15   14   13   12   11

Printed in Great Britain by CPI Antony Rowe, Chippenham and Eastbourne

Dedicated to my parents, who were always my shining light; and sister Helen, nephew Jonathan and husband Howard, who have supported me during the writing of this book.

Contents

Figures

Tables

Boxes

Foreword

What Dianne Garland has given the world in *Revisiting Waterbirth: An Attitude to Care*, a development of her previous book *Waterbirth* (Garland 1995, 2000), is a compendium of knowledge and experience that spans two decades. The continued integration of waterbirth into clinical settings around the world is in large part due to the vitality of the message that the earlier editions of this book brought to midwives and obstetricians. The use of warm water immersion has long been seen as an aid for labour, making it easier for the mother to enter into and remain in a state of hormonal bliss. In the past 20 years professionals like Dianne Garland have been reassuring mothers and midwives alike that it is safe for the baby to be born in water. Garland's experience as a hands-on midwife attending waterbirths, as well as her design and documentation of research, makes her the perfect person to lay the foundation of education for those who want to incorporate the use of water into maternity care settings.

The message in this book is simple, straightforward and very hopeful. It is hopeful in the sense that more and more women are asking how to make labour less about 'enduring the pain', and more about creating a good, healthy and loving experience of birth for the baby. Women are beginning to understand that their participation in creating a new human being is one of the most important jobs on the planet. The providers who serve those women need the encouragement that this book offers to step out of the routine medical care and become open to the possibilities that water can, indeed, change the course of a labour and should be utilized as a valuable tool for almost all women. The attitude with which professionals view a woman's ability to give birth can either enhance or detract from her experience.

Waterbirth is part of a world movement that seeks a more humane and gentler approach to childbearing. Garland has been tracking this global phenomenon for many years and includes her foreign experiences and travels so that we can see how the water connects women and their caregivers all over the planet. Dianne and I originally met 20 years ago in Kobe, Japan, at a conference where we were both speaking on waterbirth. Although we were from different sides of the pond, we shared this journey of documenting the efficacy and safety of water-birth. Our mutual passion has brought us together for conferences, workshops and presentations many times. Her excitement about demystifying waterbirth is contagious and the reader, whether midwife, doctor or mother, will experience that enthusiasm within the pages of this book.

It is my sincere desire that more US practitioners heed the message in *Revisiting Waterbirth: An Attitude to Care* and start implementing protocols in more hospitals so that all women have the opportunity to use water for labour as the best non-pharmacological pain management and to birth their babies with the ease, safety and pleasure that water so beautifully provides. On a personal note, I also hope that our tandem careers continue to bring this message to every corner of the globe. As founder and director of Waterbirth International, I have relied on Dianne Garland to provide us with a multitude of research and documentation from the UK and have used her book in its earlier editions as a teaching tool and recommended reading for nurses and midwives. I look forward to our continued collaboration in the next two decades and to using this new edition to help educate doctors, midwives and parents throughout the world.

Barbara Harper, RN, CLD, CCCE, Midwife
Founder/Director of Waterbirth International

Preface

In 1986 I was approached by a community midwife colleague to discuss the option of a mother giving birth in water. I remembered a television programme that I had seen as a student midwife in 1983 about Michel Odent in Pithiviers, showing mothers being supported to labour (and by default) birth in large paddling pools; I recall my sense of amazement at the whole scene. Sheila Kitzinger (2005) describes a similar momentous event when she visited Pithiviers in 1977.

These two influences on my embryonic career were to shape many years of work, which culminated in 2005 when I launched my own company, Midwifeexpert.com.

Why, you might ask yourself, do I start a book about waterbirth with these two references? During my career I have always tried to support colleagues and mothers with choices for care. I was relatively naive in my thinking when I believed that some 24 years later all units would be offering waterbirths and all midwives would be able to support a mother with this choice.

However, despite many international colleagues' enthusiasm and passion about this option, the situation is only very slowly moving forward. In Garland (2006c) I wrote that when I started with waterbirths in 1986 I had no vision that this would be my crusade. I write this book, *Revisiting Waterbirth: An Attitude to Care*, in the hope it will guide and support you so that you may join an international group of pioneers who steadily move forward, whether through clinical practice, research, designing birthing pools or teaching.

You may have noticed that the beginning letter of each chapter spells 'WATERBIRTH'. I have used this mnemonic to cover most of the aspects regarding the use of water and it has supported the teaching sessions that I undertake worldwide. The mnemonic was designed from lectures around the world when midwives and students identified their learning needs. It acts as a basis to discuss many aspects of waterbirth and reminds us of its many facets.

As I travel to other countries I continue to discover practitioners using water in many circumstances. These personal experiences will be highlighted throughout the text and referenced where appropriate.

Arthur Schopenuhauer (1788–1860) shared a very powerful thought regarding 'truth': 'All truth goes through three stages: first it is ridiculed, secondly it is violently opposed and thirdly it is accepted as self evident.' I am not sure where waterbirths sit within this context and possibly it depends on where you are working. Waterbirths have over the years gone through these three stages – some places have moved through all three and waterbirth is well accepted; others have got no further than ridicule.

Abbreviations

ACTH	adrenocorticotrophic hormone
AIMS	Association for Improvement in Maternity Services
APH	antepartum haemorrhage
ARM	artificial rupture of membranes
BMI	body mass index
B/P	blood pressure
CEMACH	Confidential Enquiry into Maternal and Child Health
CNST	Clinical Negligence Scheme for Trusts
COSHH	Control of Substances Hazardous to Health
CRP	C-reactive protein
CTG	cardiotocograph
DoH	Department of Health
DVT	deep vein thrombosis
EBL	estimated blood loss
FBM	fetal breathing movements
FHR	fetal heart rate
GBS	group B Streptococcus
Hb	haemoglobin
HCA	healthcare assistant
HSE	health service executive
IOL	induction of labour
IV	intravenous
LFER	lung fluid expulsion reflex
LSCS	lower segment Caesarean section
MAP	mean arterial pressure
MIDIRS	Midwives Information and Resource Service
MLU	midwife-led unit
MROP	manual removal of placenta
MRSA	methicillin-resistant Staphylococcus aureus
NHS	National Health Service
NICE	National Institute for Health and Clinical Excellence
NICU	neonatal intensive care unit
NMC	Nursing and Midwifery Council
NND	neonatal death

NSF	National Service Framework
PCT	Primary Care Trust
PCV	packed cell volume
PPH	postpartum haemorrhage
PRoM	prolonged rupture of membranes
RCM	Royal College of Midwives
RCOG	Royal College of Obstetricians and Gynaecologists
RCT	randomized control trial
RDS	respiratory distress syndrome
SB	stillbirth
SCBU	special care baby unit
SRM	spontaneous rupture of membranes
SVD	spontaneous vertex delivery
TENS	transcutaneous electrical nerve stimulator
ToP	termination of pregnancy
TOS	trial of scar
UKCC	United Kingdom Central Council
VBAC	vaginal birth after Caesarean
VE	vaginal examination
WBAC	waterbirth after Caesarean
WHO	World Health Organization

1

Professional and Governmental Support

As practising midwives in the UK we have a unique professional and governmental stance on waterbirth. Highlighted in this chapter are some of the professional and government documents that support this option. Some are more explicit (DoH 2004) than others (NICE 2007). However, when I meet people around the world the question is often raised: 'Where do I stand professionally in undertaking and supporting waterbirth?' In 2004 the Nursing and Midwifery Council (NMC) issued its latest *Midwives' Rules and Standards* within rule 6 – responsibility and sphere of practice. They wrote: 'except in an emergency a practising midwife shall not provide any care, or undertake any treatment, which she has not been trained to give'. This is often interpreted locally as meaning the midwife must undertake various educational and observational skills training before being able to participate in waterbirths. Whilst I totally agree with the principle of this statement, I find it is often used as an excuse for why a midwife cannot support a mother with this choice. The NMC does not state what type of training is required, just saying that the midwife 'must ensure she becomes competent in any new skills required for her practice'. After nearly 25 years of waterbirth practice in the UK, is this really a new skill? I would argue that it is not a new skill for the midwifery profession in the UK as a whole but may be for individual midwives. Support is vital in moving waterbirths forward and below I discuss some of the supportive mechanisms available to UK midwives. The situation is of course different in other countries and I am aware that many places do not have these benefits.

Midwifery Supervision

Supervision of midwives was written into statute in the 1902 Midwives Act; despite several later acts (1936, 1951 and 1974) this statutory obligation has basically remained unchanged. The primary purpose of supervision is to protect the public, but there can be times when there is tension between the concept of advocacy and professional care. It is required of supervisors that they provide a proactive supervision in action. With regard in particular to waterbirth, they should:

* promote childbirth as a normal, physiological event
* encourage midwives to utilize an evidence-based approach in their care delivery
* support midwives who are supporting women in making care choices
* provide additional advice to women who are experiencing difficulty in achieving their care choices
* be able to handle conflict and achieve a consensus that ensures no party feels disadvantaged.

At the present time midwifery is unique in having this statutory obligation. In 2006 the NMC published *Standards for the Preparation and Practice of Supervisors of Midwives*. Supervisors have a duty to ensure that midwives can assist mothers in their choices for labour and birth, and are there to assist in facilitating change in a challenging and changing environment.

It is outside the scope of this book to discuss supervision more fully but the role of supervisors will be explored in specific situations through this book and in Chapter 8.

Government and Professional Reports

One of the benefits of working within the National Health Service with well-established professional colleges and central government documents is that midwives are enabled to achieve standards nationally, not just locally. One such example of this is the Royal College of Obstetricians and Gynaecologists' *Safer Childbirth: Minimum Standards for the Organization and Delivery of Care in Labour* (RCOG 2007). The document focus is on woman-centred care, with an extension of the midwife's teaching role in multi-professional education. It continues with governance principles for births in all care settings (home, midwifery birth centres and consultant units) and includes a central theme of improved communication between healthcare professionals and women.

Midwives' Rules and Standards

One section of the *Midwives' Rules and Standards* (NMC 2004) continues to be relevant to waterbirths, although not exclusively so: 'Developments in midwifery care often become an integral part of the role of the midwife and may be incorporated in the initial preparation of midwives. Other developments in midwifery and obstetric practice may require that you learn new skills, but these skills do not necessarily become part of the role of all midwives.'

This is important for all midwives to review and is one of the questions raised for reflection at the end of this chapter.

National Service Framework for Children, Young People and Maternity Services

The UK Department of Health document *National Service Framework for Children, Young People and Maternity Services* (DoH 2004) (see Box 1.1) once again raised the issue of mothers having access to birthing pools, with staff who are competent to support them. Whilst similar to the Winterton Report (1992) and *Changing Childbirth* (DoH 1993), there is one fundamental difference I would like to explore.

The document states that *'all staff* [my italics] have up-to-date skills and knowledge to support women who choose to labour without pharmacological intervention, including the use of birthing pools'. The italics stress my issue. When I lecture, I ask that the host invite all vested interested parties, such as obstetricians, paediatricians, infection control etc. With a few exceptions, however, it is very rare for other disciplines to attend. I believe it is vital that when a new service is being developed,

---

Box 1.1 *National Service Framework for Children, Young People and Maternity Services* **(2004)**

NHS maternity care providers and primary care trusts ensure that:

- women have a choice of methods of pain relief during labour including non-pharmacological options
- all staff have up-to-date skills and knowledge to support women who choose to labour without pharmacological intervention, including the use of birthing pools
- access to a birthing pool, with staff competent in facilitating waterbirths, is allowed wherever possible.

all staff are involved. For example, how will support staff know the importance of thorough cleaning of a pool (especially if it looks clean) if no one has explained that 'body' fluids will have evacuated into the water even if there is no obvious blood staining? Another example would be training in emergency evacuation, using a net or hoist. Anyone who may be in the vicinity (office-based midwives) should know their role in this emergency: it may not actually be to assist with the lift, but to clear the environment or redirect help. This is further explored in Chapter 6.

Maternity Matters: Choice, Access and Continuity of Care in a Safe Service

When the Department of Health's document *Maternity Matters: Choice, Access and Continuity of Care in a Safe Service* was published in 2007 (see Box 1.2) it once again supported a mother's choice, but for me it was much more. Two paragraphs are important for the waterbirth movement. Firstly, just as women will need to realize that the choice of place of birth will influence the choice of pain relief available (for example, epidurals will only be available in certain localities), so it may be for waterbirth. In some high-risk, consultant-led units the option of waterbirth may not be practical. However, this should not be an excuse for not offering, and saying things like 'We do not have time', 'We could not stay with the mother', 'We cannot offer one-to-one care', 'We only have high-risk mothers'. These are pressures that we should challenge rather than just accept. I have even heard midwives say that they could not offer physiological third stage because they have to get women out of the labour ward within two hours. I am not trying to get political – or maybe I am – but are we really willing to accept these reasons/excuses

---

Box 1.2 *Maternity Matters: Choice, Access and Continuity of Care in a Safe Service* (DoH 2007)

- Choice of place of birth ... Women will need to understand that their choice of place of birth will affect the choice of pain relief available to them (epidurals).
- Mayday Hospital, Kent, UK ... which has three birth pools and mood lighting, has led to an increase in the number of normal births where women are giving birth with minimal pharmacological analgesia and no medical intervention.

for a low-risk choice? Are we really supporting choice and being 'with women' (which is what 'midwife' actually means)?

The second issue is about right time, right place, right people and, lastly, right leadership. Many centres have benefited from a combination of these factors, and although many have had a pool in situ for some time it is only when one factor changes that the pool seems to find a whole new lease of life. The ethos and philosophy of a department can alter dramatically when a new leader or champion arrives. It can sometimes feel like being a gladiator in the arena ready for a fight. In this situation the crowd (colleague) support is vital. This will be discussed later in Chapter 6, 'Robust Clinical Care' and Chapter 9, 'Research'.

Intrapartum Care

The document *Intrapartum Care* published by NICE (2007) stresses the importance of giving mothers the opportunity to try water labour and is another positive move forward. It is interesting, though, that it fails to mention waterbirth as such and only gives advice about water labour (see Box 1.3).

It is also heartwarming to see NICE write about physiological third stage, for so long a skill many midwives have been taught, but which is rarely used and supported. The change in direction has been mainly from midwives who believe in the physiological processes of birth. This

---

Box 1.3   Issues relevant to water from *Intrapartum Care* (NICE 2007)

This document raises several issues that are relevant to waterbirth. One-to-one care is of course not just for water labour/birth, but a gold standard for all labour/birth. I would not advocate that a mother is not supported without one-to-one care but I am very aware that sometimes we may have to balance demands of care on busy labour wards.

Women should have:
- evidence-based information
- one-to one-care
- opportunity to labour in water for analgesia
- initial, four-hourly, second stage, hourly vaginal examinations (VEs)
- physiological third stage – no early clamping
- clinical governance principles
- no pethidine < 2 hours before a bath

includes supporting mothers in having a physiological third stage. Issues surrounding this choice are discussed in Chapter 6, where I will also discuss issues of skills and dispel the myth of water emboli. Another issue raised by NICE in the guidelines is underpinning care with clinical governance principles. The seven pillars of governance (see p. 137) all sit very comfortably with water labour/birth. They support the practice that midwives who steered waterbirth through its early days were trying to encourage. These principles included multi-professional working, audit, guidelines and patient involvement. In Chapter 8 these underpinning governance principles will be further expanded.

One issue, however, that I feel I must address and challenge is regarding the timing of vaginal examinations. When supporting mothers with normal, low-risk childbirth, I personally find very little need to rely on vaginal examinations to assess progress of labour. NICE write that mothers should be offered initial, and then four-hourly and then hourly second-stage vaginal examinations. We teach midwives non-dexterous skills to assess labour; we sit with mothers and watch as their labours change during the course of the first and second stages. Whilst there is always a time and place for a vaginal examination, I believe there are other ways to assess normal labour progress. Non-dexterous skills, attitudes and intuitive behaviour are reviewed in Davis (2004), Frye (2004), Walsh (2007) and Gaskin (2008).

Our community midwife colleagues have a long history of non-dexterous skills when assessing labour at home. They utilize their skills, intuition, experience and passive skills to develop an understanding of individual mothers' labour.

Making Normal Birth a Reality

It is hoped that *Making Normal Birth a Reality* (co-authored by RCM, RCOG and NCT 2007) does not become just another rhetoric document (see Box 1.4). It identifies that even just having access to water increases the chance of a normal birth. Normal birth is facilitated by the use of water, but it is as much about our ethos, philosophy and understanding of care in labour as actually having a pool within the birth environment. I believe this was an aspect of the original use of pools at Michel Odent's unit at Pithiviers. He found women were naturally drawn to water – even running water was a powerful attraction. For many years midwives have realized that about 50 per cent of mothers leave the water before birth (personal audit data and Health Service Commission 2008). We may be able to reduce the number of mothers who leave the

---

Box 1.4   *Making Normal Birth a Reality* **(RCM, RCOG, NCT 2007)**

- Maternity commissioners, providers and NHS boards – positive focus with access to birth pools
- What increases normal birth?
- Assist in facilitating normal birth without evidence of additional risks – immersion in water.

---

water for further analgesia (not because they wish to deliver on dry land or just choice) by understanding the 'theories' of water labour and using these factors in clinical practice. Chapter 4 looks at these theories.

Towards Better Birth

This Healthcare Commission report (2008) is one of the most recent (see Box 1.5). Under the section regarding access to a pool, 95 per cent of trusts (hospitals) in the UK said that mothers had access. However, the reality of this access is often of concern: mothers are told the pool is broken, or there is no midwife who is trained, or there are not enough staff. If these same excuses were used for epidural analgesia there would be uproar (anecdotal and personal experiences). Trusts state that 11 per cent of mothers use water and seven births occur per month in a pool. Many UK birth centres can show that they achieve these numbers on their own, so the discrepancy between one unit and another is huge. Correct interpretation of this document is important for mothers and midwives so that false illusions are not created and lost opportunities do not occur. We need to address the issue of training (mentioned by the report itself), ensure the pool is available at all times, and provide care to all mothers with whichever choice of analgesia they opt for, whether that is water or something else.

Box 1.5   *Towards Better Birth* **(Healthcare Commission 2008)**

- 95% of trusts have access to birthing pools
- 11% of mothers use water
- 7 births in pool per month
- 50% of mothers leave water for delivery
- Training needs to be increased for midwives.

Education needs to be flexible, non-dogmatic, creative and proactive in its content and delivery. It should not be interpreted as 'go to a lecture, see three waterbirths, do three under supervision, then start'. You may wait a long time for these opportunities – education should always reflect individual and institutional needs (see Chapter 10, 'Teaching and Ongoing Education').

High Quality Care for All

The Darzi Report (DoH 2008) *High Quality Care for All* was published in June 2008. There are some issues within this document which again support choices for mothers. The report highlights the importance of a greater degree of control and influence over healthcare. This is important for those who find it harder to seek out services or make themselves heard. I interpret this as improving access to services for women with differing health needs (mobility issues) or women from other countries and backgrounds who do not routinely get heard when it comes to choices for labour and birth. I discuss in Chapter 5 the importance of engaging with prospective parents so that they can access information as well as direct services. Darzi goes on to say that every primary care trust (PCT) will commission 'comprehensive wellbeing and prevention services ... to meet the specific needs of their local population'. Also mentioned is the need to ensure that patients have access to clinically effective and cost-effective drugs. This issue is raised in Chapter 8.

The issue of multi-professional working will be raised throughout this book. But on the very serious side, discrepancies in practice between midwives and the medical profession was highlighted by Dingwell, cited by Alexander et al. in 1993. Although it is an old reference, I find as I travel around the world that it is still as relevant today:

> The legal process can be cruel exposure of failures in teamwork. If one professional group has adopted policies and practices at odds with those of the others, a plaintiff's lawyer will have a field day with the discrepancies. In effect, though, the objective of the tort system is to encourage good practice, so that if your practice is soundly based, the result should not be a penalty for your employer *or you*. (Alexander et al. 1993, my italics)

Kitzinger (2000) wrote: 'it seems odd that most Obstetricians seem to take more notice of a small number of babies "drowning" whilst obviously very distressing, research papers in reputable peer journals are often ignored.' Is this to do with the way that waterbirth threatens a medical perspective on labour and delivery? Is all the rhetoric surrounding waterbirths just an issue of control? Is returning choice and control to mothers a power struggle? In my experience, many countries still have little or no midwifery care and management is based on a medical model.

Fundamental to waterbirth may well be the difference between medical and midwifery staff. Whilst great movement is occurring in moving the two types of care closer together, I have found that in many other countries these two separate models of care are still in existence (see Chapter 3). The challenge for all practitioners is to work together, supporting mothers with choice and providing a safe and effective style of care.

And finally, even our titles suggest why fundamentally we work differently:

- **Obstetrician** – from Latin *obsto* 'I stand in front' (interestingly, the word 'obstacle' is derived from the same root)
- **Midwife** – 'with woman'
- **Doula** – Greek, meaning 'I serve'

Questions for Discussion and Reflection

- As a practitioner, how would you acquire the skills and attitudes required to support a mother who wishes to use water for labour and birth?
- Can you identify any areas of potential conflict in supporting a mother with this option? What processes can be utilized to assist in resolving these?

2
Why Water?

Hydrotherapy and Waterbirth History

Water has been known for its therapeutic value for many years. The Victorians were particularly known for 'taking the waters' and fashionable spa towns were built throughout the world. Water was seen as encompassing opposite ends of a continuum – stimulant versus relaxant, exercise versus rest (Inglis and West 1983).

Hydrotherapy became fashionable during the eighteenth century through Beau Nash and remained popular until the First World War. It lost its respectability and became known as a cure for insanity and of doubtful therapeutic value. Free spas disappeared by the 1940–1950s as doctors came to believe that drugs were a cure-all, although in other countries spas and therapeutic waters continued. The magnificent natural wonders of the Turkish limestone cliffs at Pamukkale still attract thousands of visitors each year. In Germany, spa towns have continued to flourish and offer early morning warm-ups, exercises, massages, loofah baths and herbal wraps!

Evidence of the use of aromatherapy and, in particular, relaxing baths can be seen in any health or pharmacy shop. Indeed, there appear to be few psychological or physical ailments that do not have their own preparation. *The Scented Bath* (Riggs 1991) is devoted to relaxation and relaxing baths. The book brings together 'twenty recipes for enchanting bathing rituals, each designed to create a certain mood, ease a specific problem or simply induce a sense of psychological and physical wellbeing'.

Thalassatherapy has developed more slowly over the past 30 years and this sea therapy includes massage, baths of differing temperatures, underwater exercises, pressurized water jets and seaweed packs. Even in today's high-tech society, the spa towns of Grofenburg in Austria and Spa in Belgium bear testimony to the use of these therapies.

So why is hydrotherapy regaining popularity? Stanway (1979) wrote:

Most often ... I feel water therapy is beneficial because it is carried out by pleasant caring people, who together with the pampered atmosphere usually surrounding the therapy, induce a sense of mental wellbeing in the patient. Mental improvement in turn produces a reduction in anxiety and stress orientated symptoms and signs and he goes away feeling better ... which is what all medicine is about.

Hydrotherapy's role in obstetrics is poorly documented, save for some references to Finnish women being taken to saunas for confinement (Nicol 1975). Chapter 4 explores theories of hydrotherapy in labour.

Waterbirth history

The earliest recorded waterbirth was in 1803, reported in France. However, there are stories of Panamanian women giving birth in water-filled hammocks, legends from the Minoans, the Chumash Native Americans in America, and from as far away as the Pacific islands including New Zealand (Napierela 1994; Wickham 2003). Other stories come from Australia, Japan, Guyana and Mongolia (Mackay 2001). In 2003 Kitzinger wrote in Wickham (2003) about the culture of waterbirth and discussed whether the accounts recalled are merely stories or whether they have any substance to them. She writes, 'waterbirth is more likely to be encountered in California, or, for that matter in Kensington, than in traditional cultures. Waterbirth is part of a new birth culture that challenges the dominant medical system of birth. It does not need to be validated by tradition.'

We have been aware that water is a powerful feminine element; indeed it is said that the ancient Greek gods used water as an eternal life giver, the priests of Egypt were delivered into water, and in the Christian faith water is used to welcome and baptize children into their religion. Mackay (2001) writes that European women travelled to the natural pools in Clach Bhan and Ben Avon in the Cairngorm mountains of Scotland, which were purported to have a powerful effect on labour pains. She describes a popular German medical book published at the turn of the twentieth century which prescribed bathing in water at body temperature, followed by a cooler bath for three minutes to assist with a difficult labour. Whether any of these 'historical' stories have any evidence can be debated but a final element is that of Aphrodite – born from the waves of the ocean and Venus. Having visited the site of her 'birth' in Cyprus (see Figure 2.1), I can vouch for its being a beautiful

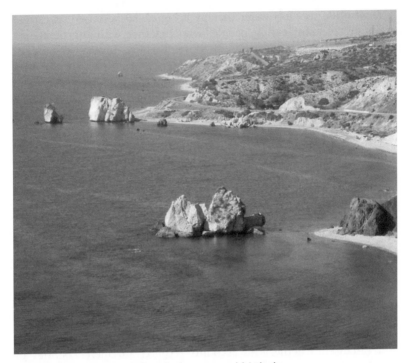

Figure 2.1 Cyprus: Aphrodite's supposed birthplace

area with waves crashing, setting sun and peace – but anything more …
well maybe I'm too pragmatic.

Harper (2005) writes about the history of waterbirth in her book
Gentle Birth Choices. She indicates that there is little concrete evidence
that any ancient cultures practised waterbirth. There appear to be
legends that the ancient Egyptians birthed selected babies under water,
and that these babies became the priests and priestess. Ancient Minoans
in Crete are said to have used a sacred temple for waterbirth, and there
are art frescoes in Minoan ruins that depict dolphins and the special
bond that many people believe we have with them as land mammals.

Harper also describes a Native American tribe, the Chumash in
central California, who were said to labour in tide pools and shallow
inlets along the beach, and continues with other references to Native
American tribes in North, Central and South America using water for
labour/birth. Finally, she records traditional stories about people in
Hawaii, Maoris from New Zealand and the Pacific people of Samoa using
water in the shallows or river environments for labour/birth.

During the course of researching this edition I was told a story by a lecturer who had been advised by Nigerian students about a particular tribe in northern Nigeria that insists that its babies are born in the local river. The community rely on fishing for their livelihood and babies born in the river are thought to be less likely to drown in later life. If the woman does not make it to the river in time for the birth, the baby is thrown into the river as soon as possible after birth to ensure that the benefits of early exposure to water can be retained.

Whether any of these stories have any substance is debatable. I do not believe they add much to the waterbirth debate, except perhaps that they reinforce what we have known for a long time: that water is a powerful relaxant during labour and birth.

However, for most practitioners in today's world the first we heard about waterbirth was from Russia and the work of Charkovsky in the early 1980s. Michel Odent came to light with his work in Pithiviers, France, also in the early 1980s, where he was using water for labour but also expanding the work of Frederick Leboyer. Leboyer (1975) wrote:

coming out into warm water, a child feels familiarity. Safe and secure, he does not breathe because he has come from water into water. When brought up to the surface his face meets the air and he breathes at last. Nestled in his mother's arms he feels security of her skin, and hears the soothing hum of her voice as she speaks words of wonder and love. He is awoken gently in this kind of environment. He opens and unfolds ... A kind, loving and gentle entry into this world.

By 1986 many practitioners around the world had started to use water as a medium for labour and birth. Making a 'splash' in the USA, Dr Michael Rosenthal, who had been inspired by Odent, was transforming his Family Birthing Center in Upland, California. In this environment he and a team of midwives/nurses provided an environment that supported women's choices in birth, and enabled an enriching birth experience for all the family. Other enlightened obstetricians took the approach that labour was best if left without inappropriate interventions, and in Keene, New Hampshire, nurses, midwives and doctors worked together to introduce both a doula programme and birthing tubs. When they presented at the 2007 Gentle Birth Conference in Portland, Oregon, they coined a phrase to explain the dramatic shift in attitudes: 'From high tech to high touch'. This is a phrase that I too have used to great advantage when explaining that waterbirth is not just about dextrous skills but about attitudes and a shift in the ethos of caring.

In the UK several practitioners were leading the way with using water. Roger Lichy, a GP in Cornwall, was able to show the first-ever waterbirth on television (*Natural Concern – Katy's Birthday*, 1988, BBC). Other pioneers included Jayn Lee Miller (who went on to create Splashdown). Information, advice and pool designs were being promoted by the Active Birth Centre and by Adam Maclean and his company Birth Pool in a Box. Whilst the commercialization of birthing pools spread, midwives were not being left behind. Ethel Burns in Oxford, Cas Nightingale at Hillingdon and of course myself in Kent were pushing the boundaries before professional and governmental bodies wrote about introducing pools (Winterton 1992 and DoH 1993).

Some of these early pioneers and references are discussed and referred to further throughout the text of this book.

Throughout the world other empowering practitioners also took the plunge. In Australia there were Dr Bruce Sutherland and Dr Andrew Davidson; and in Russia Dr Zina Bakhareva and midwife Tatyana Sargunas developed more than just home waterbirths – they pushed the boundaries by developing birth camps (see DVD listings in Chapter 11). José Luis Grefnes Sanchez and San Luis Pitosi in Mexico, Dr Geissbuhler in Switzerland and José Muscat in Malta are other notable pioneers – or mavericks, depending on your viewpoint – who have helped to develop an international network. We now know of over 100 waterbirth countries stretching from Israel to Iceland, from New Zealand to China: all four corners of the globe are now supporting parents with this choice.

Why Water for Labour and Birth?

However well prepared women are when they enter labour, major physiological and psychological changes happen. These changes may include fear, stress, pain, reduced mobility and fatigue. As long ago as the 1950s Grantly Dick-Read identified a cycle of interplay between these factors and labour outcome. Added to these factors are women's perception and expectation of labour, previous experiences (and those of others who have shared theirs) and pain tolerance threshold.

In 2009 Walsh, writing about epidurals, highlighted why he believed there is an epidemic of epidural analgesia. Some of his references are as relevant to water as to the rationale for increasing epidural rates: for example, over recent decades there has been a loss of 'rite of passage' meaning to childbirth. In a techno-rationalist society that considers pain as either preventable or treatable, a pain relief paradigm is dominant in maternity services; informed choice as an ethical imperative influences practitioners' responses to maternal requests for pain relief. I believe that despite it being 15 years since the first edition of this book, the subtitle – *An Attitude to Care* – is still as relevant as ever.

Stress in labour

Why does stress play such a part in how labour may progress? Sometimes the reaction is useful; sometimes it's a hindrance. Physical stress may occur when there is an injury – it may mean a mother will try her best to get away from trauma by changing position. Psychological stress, which causes an increase in adrenaline, noradrenaline and catecholamines, prompts the labouring mother to seek assistance – the birth companion's role. Every woman is individual and it is that individuality which allows many to adapt to the environment of labour and return to a normal balanced situation. See the section on normal adaptive process in Chapter 4.

Just as I have said that each mother should be treated as an individual, so should the baby. Can this be related to the clinical picture? How often as midwives are we confronted with apparent 'fetal compromise', which at delivery is not borne out by the Apgar scores or cord pH and is unrelated to neonatal problems? This is not to say we should be complacent with regard to fetal compromise but just that we should be aware of the fine interplay between mother and fetus. This is explored further in Chapter 4.

Pain in labour

Pain results from intense stimuli, which may cause or threaten to cause tissue damage. The pain receptors respond to these stimuli and assist in avoiding or minimizing bodily damage. We know that if pain occurs during labour then there is a rise in catecholamines and corticosteroids, with a potential to cause maternal acidosis and a reduction in uterine activity.

Reduced mobility in labour

Reduction in mobility in labour has two main causes. Firstly, it becomes increasingly difficult to move when on dry land, and secondly, modern obstetric practice inhibits mothers through bed design, electronic monitoring and interventions. Some efforts have been made with telemetry monitoring and 'mobile' low-dose epidurals. On the midwifery front, numerous birthing aids have been designed – stools, balls, chairs and supportive hanging birth devices. These can help a mother to remain upright and mobile during her labour. Any reduction in mobility causes potential problems: no gravity, vena caval compression and inherent risk of maternal hypotension, and reduced placental blood flow.

Fatigue in labour

As labour progresses the woman will experience a degree of reduced gastrointestinal absorption and dehydration as gastric emptying is slowed and reserves are utilized in labour (Davison et al. 2005; Pairman et al. 2006; O'Sullivan et al. 2009). This maybe compounded where the woman is unable to eat and drink. Throughout the world there are many hospitals where practice does not allow mothers to eat or drink, and in order to neutralize gastric contents an oral preparation is given (ranitidine hydrochoride).

The debate about eating and drinking in labour continues (O'Sullivan et al. 2009). The summary of this randomized controlled trial (RCT) said: 'eating during labour did not influence neonatal or obstetric outcomes, including rates of spontaneous and operative delivery or duration of labour'. This is the consensus opinion of *Intrapartum Care* (NICE 2007).

There is, of course, a plethora of anatomy and physiology books which can assist in underpinning some of these issues (see Coad and Dunstall 2005; Stables and Rankin 2005; Wylie 2005).

Advantages and Disadvantages of Water in Labour

Having reviewed anecdotal work from practitioners and mothers, I list the advantages and disadvantages below as a summary of their comments. In each category I have listed the maternal and then midwifery issues:

- **Advantages of using water**
  o choice/control in labour and delivery
  o pleasant relaxing environment
  o increased acceptance of 'normality'

o drug-free environment
o non-interventionist approach to care
o positive clinical outcomes (see Chapter 9, 'Research')
o ? long-term neonatal development (this has not been studied and the comment is from observation only – claims are made that these children develop physically and psychologically better, but the only study is Smirnov (2002); see Chapter 9)
o regaining 'traditional' skills
o increased liaison/communication with mother
o staff recruitment – attracts staff to unit
o attracts clients
o good PR for unit – high profile
o income generation – pool hire

• **Disadvantages of using water**
o cost of tub hire or facilities
o client selection – some women excluded
o 'elitist'
o physiological issues – some women not successful
o clinical issues – negative outcomes (PPH)
o midwife education – support and teaching required
o standard setting – defining normality
o midwife outcomes – personal philosophy/injury

Water assists the physiological process: it comforts and warms the mother, cradles her during contractions, allows her to descend into her own zone and, by improving mobility and encouraging an upright position, allows descent of the fetal head. Non-intervention is standard. Just sitting and being a passive observer, a midwife practises skills and intuition to the point of knowing when to remain passive and, more importantly, when to act. In this environment there is no clinical indication to intervene with intrusive technology – no cardiotocograph, no artificial rupture of membranes, no routine use of oxytocics, and intervention only when the clinical situation warrants it. The environment is supportive both physically – warm, deep water soothing over a mother's abdomen may reduce pain and relax muscles, and reduce pressure on muscles and ligaments and enable her to move around the pool – and psychologically – from midwives who as skilled practitioners understand the 'watch and wait' approach. We encourage, guide and support the mother through this normal process of childbirth. Finally, water enables a mother to feel empowered because she is in control, has the ability to move around the pool, change positions and feel relaxed in her own regression. For some mothers, this empowerment has meant a lot of investment in time and/or money in seeking out this watery option – how satisfying that must feel during labour!

The widespread introduction of the use of water during the early 1980s has seen a resurgence over the past few years. Indeed, the use of water is now included in most maternity services guidelines, as an adjunct to non-pharmacological forms of analgesia. Whilst most service documents do not explore a woman's motivation for using water, government documents have once again raised the response levels for service providers to act on the demand for the use of water. The Winterton Report (1992) and *Changing Childbirth* (DoH 1993) raised the bar by stating that units should aim to provide a water labour/birth service. Unfortunately, it appears that many units could not or would not accept the challenge of water labour/birth and only a few enlightened units around the UK supported this choice for mothers. Even when the UKCC (UK Central Council for Nursing, Midwifery and Health Visiting) wrote in 1994 that waterbirths 'fall within the duty of care and *normal* [my italics] practice of a midwife', it never really became mainstream. By 2004 the *National Service Framework* said that 'women have a choice of methods of pain relief during labour including non-pharmacological options' (DoH 2004). This was followed by *Maternity Matters* (DoH 2007). Further reports in 2007 and 2008 have continued with their support.

Research Relevant to Practice

There is a small body of research which has attempted to identify the decision-making experience of mothers who wish to use water in their labour/birth. Wu and Chung (2003) undertook a small study to interview mothers wishing to use water, who were then interviewed mainly at home. Four themes were reflected throughout this study: (a) that women were dissatisfied with current medical care (because they feel manipulated and controlled in hospital); (b) they had experienced negative previous delivery experiences; (c) women consulted their relatives for opinion and support; and (d) many attempted to achieve their goal by persuasion or just chose not to tell family about their plans.

Comment: Whilst it was only a small study (nine mothers), the authors comment that they believe these mothers were reflective of the general maternity population. As a midwife I may find the size of the study difficult to justify in terms of total population; however, as a waterbirth midwife, I can identify with the themes. Indeed, they are often identified when I discuss with mothers their motivation to use water (see Chapters 5 and 9).

One of the most interesting issues in the waterbirth debate was raised by Gould (2007) in discussing why water is often difficult to introduce into mainstream (apologies for the pun) care on labour wards. She writes that this is because we have made water so complicated, with our criteria, guidelines and 'training', that midwives are afraid to make the transition from normal bathing in labour (well known by our older midwives) to the 'all singing, all dancing' birthing pools now on the market. Where water is well supported in the right environment it is accepted not just by midwives but also by the diversity of mothers within our care. I have always stressed during my lectures that mothers should not be made to jump through hoops to use water, attending specific classes, 'signing up' to using the pool only if certain midwives are on duty or (in the worst-case scenario) being denied because midwives are too busy. If we provide labour care and part of our support is use of an analgesic – whether in water or in the form of an epidural – we should be able to support a mother in any birthing environment. If we are too busy to support a mother with water labour, are we also too busy to offer an epidural? Providing care for mothers should ensure we can offer all choices. I would far rather have a mother in a pool with minimal 'risks' than the inherent risks of a mother with an epidural (hypotension/pyrexia/slow progress and continuous monitoring). In scenarios where this negative attitude to care still prevails, we should support each other and challenge those colleagues who fail to provide this option. I am sure that there would be a clinical risk form produced if a midwife failed to support a mother with an epidural because she was too busy!

Maternity Matters (DoH 2007) drew attention to the fact that mothers may need to recognize that all options may not be available in all care settings. The example they highlight is that an epidural will not be available in all care settings (home or birth centre), but maybe we should also stress this to mothers regarding water pools. In high-risk labour wards the option of a pool may not be possible: it may be a case of 'right time, right place, and right staff'.

'Greek goddess' scenario

The 'Greek goddess' scenario was coined in the 1980s when it became apparent to practitioners that many mothers believed water to be the panacea for all evils. Women seemed to think that if they entered a pool there would be no problems and they would have a wonderful birth experience. The reality is far more practical: in my experience, only half the mothers who enter water will labour in the pool and of those only a third will stay in and deliver. There are also huge variations in accessibility to water pools around the UK and abroad. So mothers who wish for this option may find their desire challenged by the availability or otherwise of a pool.

When a woman approaches me about this option, I always ask what attracts her to using water during labour and birth. Sometimes she may highlight a poor previous birth experience, so it is important to review her medical records if possible. Then we can go step by step through the records to assess the impact technology/interventions had on outcomes. We can then write a birth plan, and options for labour and delivery that fulfil two main aims – safety and realistic expectations. In some situations we may need to challenge basic assumptions of care, such as continuous monitoring or eating and drinking in labour (see Chapter 3).

Dolphin care

In *Beyond the Blue* (Cochrane and Callen 1998) the relationship beyond land and sea mammals is explored. The dolphin 'midwife' and 'teacher' is discussed, together with the mammal's unique ability to receive subtle energy forces around them. This telepathy may be the reason why we, as land mammals, are attracted to the sea for its healing properties. In Victorian times 'taking the waters' was a common practice and even now people tend to head to the sea for their holidays.

There has been some work on the 'dolphin' concept – originally highlighted by the early work of Igor Charkovsky and Michel Odent (Sidenbladh 1983; Odent 1998) This work of labouring/birthing with dolphins is almost seen as a spiritualistic rite of passage. It is thought that we as humans have a strong bond with sea mammals, especially dolphins. Whilst not widely accepted in the UK, this concept is still supported in some parts of the world.

Some of the original concepts from Charkovsky, including his initial introduction to water, have recently been reproduced on the internet.

When his daughter was born very pre-term, he believed that by using water he could reduce her oxygen demands and that the weightlessness would reduce the 'shock' of gravity on the newborn's brain. Charkovsky is seen either as a genius, saviour and talented scientist or as someone whose approach is barbaric, with his baby water yoga. If you wish to read Charkovsky's full story then I suggest you read Sidenbladh (1983). Elena Tonetti continued the work with her 'conscious water birth' movement in Russia and now lives in the USA.

It is important, however, to remember that 'dolphin therapy' is developing around the world, from the United States to New Zealand. This work is using the sonic attributes that dolphins are believed to have and the strong attraction and healing properties they possess.

For most mothers this concept is only taken as far as having dolphin music playing in the pool room.

Regression/zoning out

Several authors have written about the healing power of water transcending to another level with rebirthing (Star 1986). Water can certainly assist mothers to regress and I have seen this for myself. In *Ideal Birth* (Ray 1986) Ray describes spiritual rebirthing, and pre-pregnancy or labour regression, when a mother uses this technique to 'zone out' or regress into her own 'space'. Today this is seen as similar to hypnobirthing.

Women often express – and midwives see in practice – a degree of 'regression'. This is well described in the first waterbirth that I experienced in 1987. Dawn wrote that she felt she was floating away, still aware of our presence as midwives but not intruding in her watery world. Her lagoon experience formed a concept in my mind of a physiological regression, but not drug induced, albeit the descriptions are very similar. Nowadays, regression tanks are being used for post-traumatic stress disorder; perhaps there something we can learn from this process.

Taoist philosophy often uses the powerful quality of water as a metaphor for human experiences. It allows a 'flowing' balance both physically and psychologically that gives resistance and support.

There is a resurgence in water therapies in watsu (a form of body massage). A new company called Water Journeys explores these thoughts and allows the individual to move into deep areas of relaxation and self-awareness.

Research Relevant to Practice

Richmond (2003) wrote about a small audit of 189 mothers who experienced waterbirth. In this study the results showed that waterbirth is a consumer-led trend, mainly pursued by middle-class women – see Chapter 5, 'Engaging with Parents'. Mothers said that they felt waterbirth offered a drug-free, gentle birth choice and that in water they would feel more in control. Mothers perceived waterbirth as therapeutic. Results showed that there were no significant behaviour differences between waterborn and non-waterborn babies. Mothers' descriptions suggested their babies were more alert, more peaceful, calmer, less stressed, but in statistical tests no significant differences were shown.

Comment: Although only a small study, this highlights an interesting disparity between what is documented and what is reported to midwives, and what we see in clinical experience. In my professional experience, I have seen how quiet water babies are at birth; they star gaze and have a tendency not to cry immediately. Mothers with whom I have maintained contact say that their waterbabies are quieter and calmer than previous children born on dry land. However, it is difficult to say whether this is based on a positive birth experience or on actual differences with the baby.

The list in Box 2.1 gives a summary of perceived benefits of using water based on personal experience, studies (Balaskas and Gordon 1992;

Box 2.1   Perceived psychological benefits of using water

- floatation sensation
- improved experience of pregnancy, labour and delivery
- increased self-control/altered consciousness
- increased pain threshold
- increased receptiveness to baby
- increased mother and baby interaction
- reduced fear and anger
- secure, warm, private and quiet environment
- pleasurable/reassuring serene effect
- symbolic relationship/regression
- familiar supportive staff
- increased emotional experience for caregivers

Beech 1996; Hall and Holloway 1998; Buckley 2005; Harper 2005; McCandlish and Page 2006, to name but a few) and consumer articles (Bailey 2009; Stockton 2009; Craig 2010). It is based on 'perceived' benefits since many have not been scientifically researched.

Safe and secure environment

Women often seek water as a means to provide them with a safe, secure environment. In the UK this is not as remote an idea nor unlikely as you might think: rising infection rates (MRSA) and LSCS rates make hospitals unsafe, in many women's eyes. In other parts of the world the environment for birth is not conducive to safe and secure delivery, and birth may leave the mother traumatized. Two films which were released in 2007/8 – *The Business of Being Born* and *Orgasmic Birth* – showed the public at large how birth could be peaceful and calm away from a medicalized situation (see Chapter 11 for details).

Women recall the safe and secure environment of water that they may have experienced to deal with other times in their lives (during dysmenorrhoea, say, or jet lag or stressful situations). Water now draws on those times and provides a calm and familiar environment for labour and birth.

Michel Odent's revolutionary care at Pithiviers was aimed at empowering mothers and increasing the physiological components of labour and birth (reducing adrenergic secretions, promoting endorphin production and reducing sensory input). He wrote (Odent 1984): 'Water can be as comforting as a lover, a mother or a midwife.'

Sarah Buckley, author of *Gentle Birth, Gentle Mothering* (2005), writes about her own personal waterbirth when her baby, Jacob, was born at home in water, with her family around her. She describes how although with doctor, midwife, children and husband around her the room seemed rather full, the pool allowed her some 'private space'. She finishes with the words, 'waterbirth provides a safe, satisfying and gentle start for mother and baby'.

Non-interventionist

On questioning mothers, one of the most frequent comments is, 'In the water no one can interfere with my labour.' Well, in a purist sense this is true. However, what can be done on dry land can also be done in water; there are examples world-wide of interventions occurring in water (cannulation, episiotomy, oxytocic use, ventouse, spinals and continuous monitoring). All practitioners who are performing these interventions may feel they can justify their actions (and of course one would sincerely hope they can), but one might wonder whether this is about remaining in control, not being able to let go of modern-day concepts of care. The concepts of waterbirth and technology really are in conflict: medical versus midwifery models, active versus passive management of care. I believe that where these interventions exist they should be challenged. See the section in Chapter 3 on challenges to practice.

Mothers who choose to use water often do so in order to avoid these interventions and should be prepared to challenge if they are introduced. Informed choice and not informed compliance is the order of the day. Mothers are seeking a physiological labour and birth; water supports this with low interventions, safe care and skilled practitioners.

Research Relevant to Practice

Katz et al. (1990) undertook a small study comparing bed rest with immersion in water for oedema in pregnancy. The study had three treatments for oedema: supine bed rest, sitting in a bathtub of waist-deep water (32 °C) and sitting in shoulder-deep water at 32 °C. Measurements were taken of reduction in mean arterial pressure, sodium clearance, creatinine and total protein levels. Shoulder-deep immersion produced the greatest decline in MAP (mean arterial pressure). All other markers were similar.

Conclusion: immersion appears to be a safe and more rapid method than bed rest to mobilize extravascular fluid during pregnancy.

Comment: This was only a small study of 11 women – however, repeating this study would be invaluable. The psychological benefits for mothers of not being restricted to bed rest is not explored although conservative management today would probably not include long periods of bed rest.

Of course, not all publicity adds professional support to the water-birth movement and the issue of non-intervention often quoted by mothers as the reason for wishing to use water. In 2001 an article by Sumpter highlighted some of the problems she encountered when seeking to have a non-interventionist birth (I should add she was also keen to have a non-interventionist pregnancy). The reason I mention this mother's story is mainly because of the heading of the article, which is

---

Box 2.2 Perceived physiological benefits of using water

- increased relaxation
- increased pelvic diameters
- improved contractions
- increased endorphins and oxytocin production/gate control theory
- increased oxygen and blood supply
- increased peripheral/muscle/skin temperature
- decreased pain
- increased skin stimuli – change in pain
- perception – increased hormone production
- relaxation of perineal tissues
- increased velocity of nerve conduction
- decreased gravity
- decreased pressure on vena cava
- decreased pressure on abdominal muscles/joints/ligaments

'Waterbirth mother accused of illegal birth and child neglect'. It makes sobering reading. Unfortunately, I still hear of mothers being bullied into care that is not their choice (often with little or no medical rationale); more of that in Chapter 3 when I discuss criteria for use.

Mothers often choose water because they feel that they will maintain power and avoid intervention, medicalization and a cascade of intervention – not always resulting in a LSCS (lower segment Caesarean section) but from a mother's perspective a poor birth experience. Just because a mother has a vaginal birth, it does not mean that she has had a normal physiological labour and birth, nor a satisfying psychological delivery.

Box 2.2 lists some of the perceived physiological benefits of water (the same authors listed above for Box 2.1 may help you to expand this work).

Reduced pathology

Water is very beneficial to mothers who may have a small degree of pathology (see Box 2.3), in particular those who have raised blood pressure which has been correctly diagnosed as essential hypertension or pregnancy-induced hypertension. Women with either of these blood pressure problems can benefit from the physiological hypotension that occurs when they enter the water. They need careful monitoring to ensure that the blood pressure does not compromise them or their baby – highly unlikely, but you may wish to adapt how often you record the blood pressure. I have had experience of both these scenarios, the blood pressure and fetal heart rate auscultated taken every 15 minutes for the

---

Box 2.3   Changes to interventions/decreased 'pathology' when using water

- reduced blood pressure
- increased diuresis
- decreased adrenaline and noradrenaline
- reduced production of catecholamines – stress/dysfunctional labour
- decreased pain perception
- reduced use of other analgesics
- reduced augmentation
- increased removal of waste products
- reduced energy use to maintain upright position

---

first 2 hours following immersion. This was based on intuition, clinical skills and a little research.

The other group of women who would benefit are those with a high BMI (body mass index). The Archimedes principle allows 75 per cent of weight reduction once in the water. This would benefit women who have high BMI and all them to be more mobile than on dry land. However, in many hospitals/birth centres they are excluded from using the pools, and yet they would probably benefit greatly from using water in labour. The 2003–5 CEMACH report identifies that mothers with a BMI of 35+ do have more complex labour outcomes. They are currently undertaking a study to identify factors which have an impact and outcomes for these mothers. I believe these mothers require individual risk assessment (see Chapter 3).

Harper (2005) cites Katz regarding the physiological effect that water has after 20–30 minutes of immersion. They describe the notable redistribution of blood volume, which stimulates the release of atrial natriuretic peptide (ANP) by specialized heart cells. There is a close and complex relationship between the natriuretic peptide system and the activity of the posterior pituitary gland, producing more oxytocin.

One-to-one care/autonomy of midwife

In some countries midwives are utilizing water labour/birth as a means to regain their professional autonomy. Medical staff (with some exceptions – Ponnette, Rosenthal, Odent, Muscat etc.) are often unwilling or unable to be passive caregivers to mothers who wish to labour in pools. Often, in my experience, they find it inconceivable that as midwives we may 'appear to stand by and do nothing'. Of course, what I believe we

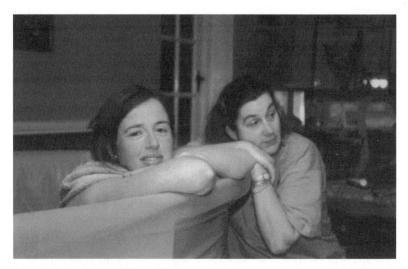

Figure 2.2   Masterly inactivity

are doing is acting in a watchful, masterly environment of inactivity, ready to act if required (see Figure 2.2).

I purposely write of 'practitioners' and not just 'midwives', as in many countries there are other colleagues who offer water and have embraced the concepts of water. In Keene, New Hampshire, doctors, labour nurses and midwives work cohesively to support mothers with this option, using their 'high tech to high touch' concept of care. In Ostend, Belgium, midwives and doctors and aquanatal teachers have developed the aquatic experience. Their collaborative efforts have led to a very empowering birth environment.

There does appear to be a suggestion emitting from certain quarters that mothers choose water to ensure that they receive one-to-one care. They seem to believe that because there is 'training' involved and competency packages and they know that only certain midwives do waterbirths, they will be able to receive almost elitist care and avoid being left on their own during labour. With current pressures on labour wards mothers may be opting for waterbirth for reasons of one-to-one care rather than as a choice for pain relief or birth (Miller and Magill-Cuerden 2006). In the NICE 2007 *Intrapartum Care* guidelines the concept of one-to-one care in labour is written as a key priority for implementation of the guidelines. It is a reality check for many practitioners that whilst these national guidelines are once again identifying one-to-one care as a key priority, mothers choose water because they believe that is the one way to ensure they receive what is required. Often water is used in midwife-led care units or home birth and enhances one-to-one care. As this style of care becomes mainstream it may improve staffing levels in consultant units.

Newborn

Wielder (1999) writes that water is a healer: we are nourished in it for 9 months, born into it, return to it to relax, play and exercise. We are baptized in water, made up (as newborns) of 99 per cent water, drink it to survive and use it to cleanse ourselves.

What is interesting is the very natural attraction that we have as land mammals to water. It is worth considering that some practitioners believe we had an aquatic development period in our evolution. A 3-day-old fetus is 97 per cent water, and by 8 months 81 per cent. Even as adults a high percentage of our bodies is made up of water – 50–70 per cent.

Children, of course, can recognize the value of water and it is wonderful to see a newborn baby swimming naturally long before it can crawl or walk. I witnessed this in Israel in 2008 and the ethos of the water education offered there can be read about in Chapter 10.

A final note: I am always amazed at the diversity of countries and care settings where waterbirths are supported – in high-rise flats, old and new houses, old and new hospitals, boats and tents. They all have two things in common: skilled and knowledgeable practitioners and a clean, readily available supply of water.

Rosenthal (1991) wrote:

Warm water immersion can best be understood in this context ... which views birth as a normal biological process, not as an illness or procedure ... thus the practitioner who embraces this approach should be prepared to play a secondary role in childbirth, informing women of their options and supporting their decisions.

Questions for Discussion and Reflection

- What makes a woman choose water as against another form of analgesia?
- Think through what benefits you have seen/experienced when mothers use water.

3
Accentuating Normality

We are educated to support normality and recognize deviations from the norm and, where appropriate, summon medical aid throughout pregnancy, labour and birth.

As midwives – and particularly at this time – we are being encouraged to promote normality and particularly the worldwide aim of reducing the Caesarean section rate. How does waterbirth support these issues? Two UK government documents, the *National Service Framework for Children, Young People and Maternity Services* (DoH 2004) and *Maternity Matters* (DoH 2007), have raised questions surrounding the use of water to promote normality. However, in this chapter many facets of normality will be explored, including challenging normal midwifery practice and regaining traditional midwifery skills.

Waterbirth promotes the natural and normal physiological process of birth. Its non-intervention, non-pharmacology analgesia and midwifery model of care all support this attitude. As midwives we experience and explore the normal ebbs and flows of labour. There is an underlying belief with waterbirth practitioners that labour and birth *is a normal physiological process, that women have the ability to give birth with skilled practitioners and water can act as an adjunct to this process.*

In this chapter will also explore some of the reasons why midwives feel threatened and unconfident with water for labour and delivery, and suggest strategies for dealing with the confidence and competence issues.

Midwifery or Medical Model of Care

To start, however, it is vital to raise the issue of normal midwifery skills and attitudes. As student midwives we learn how to enhance labour, support mothers with choices and develop skills and attitudes which will give us confidence in the birth environment. However, one thing that continues to give concern, in my personal experience, is that midwives around the world are not 'permitted' to utilize these skills in restrictive labour wards – therefore the expansion of midwife-led units (sadly not home births) in the UK. In this environment midwives can use their skills, develop confidence – and importantly, competence – in normal basic care (this will be further discussed in Chapter 6, 'Robust Clinical Care'). In 2007 Clift-Matthews wrote about the ability of midwives to take this responsibility, acquire confidence and competence and use their intuition.

If we do not permit midwives to broaden their skills they feel disempowered and the cycle of disenchantment with our role is perpetuated. Banks (2009) continues with this theme from New Zealand, writing that 'waterbirth represents a past and present struggle to practice midwifery in a society that embraces technology and medical interventions throughout the childbearing continuum – a value system which poses threats to the midwifery profession (and childbearing women) in New Zealand (sadly not just in New Zealand but world wide)'.

I should add that I believe there is a fundamental difference between midwives' and obstetricians' attitudes to childbirth around the world. Whilst we have different skills – and obstetricians are vital when a deviation from the norm occurs – in personal correspondence and visits I have witnessed a vast difference in practice. As midwives we can have a fundamental impact on labour by the way that we care and 'manage' labour. Table 3.1 shows, in a simplistic way, the differences in the two models of care worldwide.

On a personal level, I believe that many midwives have an inbuilt belief in the mother's ability to give birth, whereas medical staff often only view labour and birth as normal in retrospect. Even our two titles bear the hallmarks of the differences between the professions. 'Obstetrician' is derived from the Latin *obsto* 'I stand in front'. 'Midwife', on the other hand' means 'with woman'. Maybe this fundamental issue can shed light upon why two professionals have such different attitudes.

Table 3.1 The medical and midwifery models

Medical model	*Midwifery model*
Active management of labour	Non-intervention
Hormonal infusions	Support with birth companions
High use of technology	Complementary therapies
Hospital clinical environment	Comfortable home-like environment

Brook (1976), writing about midwives, states:

> Midwives' work was based on belief in the evidence of the senses. She trusted, and the pregnant woman trusted in her, ways to deal with the hazards of pregnancy and childbirth ... that midwives were viewed as witches as it was claimed they had magical powers [well!!] ... simply because they were well versed in the healing properties of herbs and used them medically.

Benko (2009) writes about choice for mothers in using water, particularly high-risk mothers who often have less options available to them and yet may well benefit from the physiological and psychological benefits of water. She discusses high-risk mothers (high BMI, hypertension, previous LSCS and diabetes). There is a need to work multi-professionally to standardize guidelines, giving consideration to health and safety, infection control and evidence-based practice. Many units and practitioners have been undertaking this for many years, which has led to guidelines, care pathways (especially for high-risk mothers – see the section below on VBAC) and working together for mothers and babies. As *Maternity Matters* (DOH 2007) states, the medical profession needs to 'work together in the best interest of women and babies, enabling them to achieve the positive and satisfying birth experience expected by today's parents'.

Criteria for Use of Water for High-risk Mothers

Vaginal birth after Caesarean section (VBAC) and group B streptococcus (GBS) infection are probably the two most talked-about subjects and the ones that women request information on.

Vaginal birth after Caesarean section

Four main factors that are extremely important in the safe and effective use of water for VBAC mothers are: (1) risk of scar dehiscence, usually quoted as 0.5–1 per cent (NICE 2004); (2) appropriate skills of midwives and doctors in dry-land VBAC; (3) skills in waterbirth; and (4) risk assessment process.

A plethora of information has been recorded on scar rupture over the past few years. Guise et al. (2004) report that trial of labour has an increased risk of rupture of 2.7 per cent, whereas the most successful results occur with spontaneous onset of labour. Indeed, in the UK many obstetricians will not consider induction of labour with a mother following LSCS. It is possible with the right environment, support and risk assessment to support these mothers wishing to use water. I myself published such a system in Garland (2006b). It is important always to evaluate the rate of Caesarean sections in light of changes to demography (higher BMI ratios and older first-time mothers) (Leitch and Walker 1998; Kiran and Jayawickrama 2002).

Research Relevant to Practice

In 2008 Sellar reported on an MLU (midwife-led unit) in Fife, Scotland, looking at their experience of VBAC and water labour/birth. Whilst not such a comprehensive selection/assessment was used as in Garland (2006b), 27 women were deemed able to have had a normal midwife package of care. The results showed no repeat LSCS and 10 mothers had waterbirths.

The labour durations showed no difference; perineal trauma and Apgars were the same as normal delivery. The service was given a positive feedback by mothers. Sellar also comments that in many areas of the UK the management of VBAC under a medical model would be resistant to the use of water.

The culture of midwifery does not always support the mavericks of our profession, those midwives who have pushed the boundaries, for example Caroline Flint and Ina May Gaskin. They should be supported to work positively and be proactive in change. In 2006 I wrote about the VBAC work being undertaken in a district general hospital in Kent, England. A risk assessment was undertaken with full and informed involvement of mothers who had had previous LSCS to audit whether water was a safe and realistic option for these mothers. Although it was only a small audit, the results, I believe, were impressive; mothers expressed a real interest in the opportunity to participate. See the section on criteria risk assessment below.

'Out of criteria clinics': in one London hospital a specialist clinic is run for any mother who is seeking 'out of criteria' care. This may be for home, water or birth centre delivery. There are other centres offering a similar service which are run by very experienced midwives working alongside mothers.

In support of midwives who facilitate water VBAC, Bailey (2009) wrote about a mother who had a home waterbirth following four previous Caesarean sections. This is a remarkable story to read and shows that with the right support and the skills and knowledge of midwives, a powerful and positive outcome is achievable. This is particularly beautiful since the article was by a midwife who has a wonderful birth practice in Hawaii and, as she says, 'I have been blessed to serve many women in three different countries since 1986.'

VBACs may gain a new name if water is encouraged for use with previous Caesarean section mothers: WBAC (waterbirth after Caesarean). Davies (2009) writes that the benefits of using water – improved uterine perfusion, decreased pain perception, shorter labours, decreased augmentation and reduced maternal anxiety – are all factors which may offer advantages to women labouring with a scarred uterus. Davies, like many other authors, says that monitoring the maternal pulse whilst in labour (and maybe antenatal and early intrapartum) may give a good marker regarding scar dehiscence (serous fluid leak will cause peritoneal irritation, shock response and increased pulse rate).

In Ostend, Belgium, Ponette and his team started using water for the types of mothers and babies whom other practitioners might consider high risk. Indeed, twins, breech and VBAC mothers are now using the pools using their own strict criteria and monitoring (scans, FHR monitoring, CT scans and pelvic diameter measurements). They do have exclusions for water use: namely when an IV (intravenous) oxytocin drug is required or heavy sedation is needed (presumably epidural).

Care pathway suggestion for VBAC mothers

Figure 3.1 shows an example of a care pathway that I established several years ago for mothers wishing to use water after a previous Caesarean section. The two main parameters for this were safety and realistic expectation. I have to stress that the midwives were skilled in waterbirths and supported a low-risk attitude to risk-assessed mothers for VBAC. It was also multi-professional and the obstetricians worked with midwives to design this care plan. Needless to say, it was also audited (Garland 2006b).

An issue which is commonly raised with VBAC mothers using water concerns continuous monitoring, although you can see that in the care plan in Figure 3.1 that has been shown not always to be required. Interestingly, the Royal Australian and New Zealand College of Obstetricians and Gynaecologists (2008) write in their guidelines (under normal care, not VBACs or other high-risk mothers) that 'management problems created by water immersion in labour ... continuous foetal

---

Care pathway for VBAC mothers

Initially
- Mother contacts Trust lead for VBAC
- Information gained from mother as to options available for VBAC
- Informed consent to obtain old obstetric records
- Discussion re low-risk VBAC – scar dehiscence (1:100–200)
- Motivation for using water established
- Attend specific classes/contact VBAC support group

- Initial risk assessment by consultant obstetrician/midwife

- Form (this chart) signed and copy sent to mother and hospital records

On admission – no envisaged or actual problems
- Admission observations and CTG normal
- Vaginal examination to confirm cervix 3–4 cm (established labour or as individually discussed and recorded with mother)

- Hydrotherapy – as per Trust guidelines

- CTG and vaginal examination to assess progress of labour – 4-hourly:

Labour progressing
CTG normal

Labour not progressing
CTG abnormal

Return to pool
Repeated every 4 hours whilst in labour

Return to dry land care

Mother asked to leave water for delivery

If the mother does not leave the water for birth and in the midwives' clinical judgement this is a realistic option, the decision must be documented and the senior midwife on duty informed of rationale.

Active third stage is advised on dry land.

Figure 3.1 Care pathway for VBAC mother (adapted from Garland 2006b)

monitoring is only possible using telemetry and that foetal surveillance is limited to intermittent auscultation.'

The NICE *Intrapartum Care* guidelines (2004) do recommend electronic fetal heart rate monitoring (interestingly, the word 'continuous' is not documented). In these care settings units should have access to

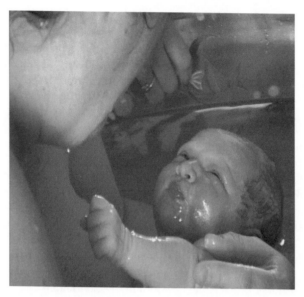

Figure 3.2   VBAC mother at home – Imogen meets her mother, Linda

Caesarean section, immediate blood transfusion and data information on risk rates for scar rupture.

On a personal level, I believe that mothers who have had a previous LSCS need to have belief and faith in their ability to give birth vaginally (depending, of course, on the reason why the LSCS was undertaken). As practitioners we need to ensure a process as shown in Figure 3.1 is designed, and be watchful, patient, skilled and also support the mother's ability to give birth. Figure 3.2 shows a happy outcome for a VBAC mother.

Group B streptococcus infection

This is one criterion which causes a dilemma when opting for a water labour/birth. There are ways to support a mother with GBS infection, bearing in mind estimates that indicate 25 per cent of labouring mothers will be carrying GBS. Easmon (1986) and the GBS Society information group highlight the fact that although it is the most common life-threatening infection in a newborn in the UK (Heath et al. 2004), group B streptococcus infection is still a relatively uncommon problem. Heath et al. stress that 99 per cent of babies do not have a problem even though their mothers are carrying GBS. Most babies are exposed to GBS when the membranes rupture and during vaginal birth; they are colonized and remain well, with only a very few developing early onset GBS infection. In the UK this equates to 0.5–3.6 per cent per 1000 babies (Centres for Disease Control and Prevention 2002). We believe, therefore, that babies maybe be 'colonized but not compromised'.

Research Relevant to Practice

The only report on the effects of using water in the presence of group B streptococcus was published in 2006 by Zanetti-Dallenbach et al. This study in Switzerland reviewed swab results from antenatal mothers (taken at 37–40 weeks from vagina and rectum), neonatal swabs from umbilicus and pharynx, and bath water used for labour/delivery.

There was a higher concentration of GBS colonization from the water than from the delivery bed (65% versus 25%). However, interestingly, the waterbirth babies showed less acquisition of GBS (19% versus 31%), perhaps suggesting that there is a 'wash-out effect' with waterbirth that protects the newborn from colonization.

Some mothers have been offered waterbirth with antibiotics. The vein is cannulated to give the antibiotics and the cannula removed before the woman enters the water. If a second dose is required, she has to be recannulated. However, over the past few years mothers have discovered that clindamycin is only required 8-hourly. There may be cost implications if this drug is used (see Table 3.2).

On a personal level, I have heard of a unit that is trialling oral antibiotics for the management of GBS.

RCOG (2003) guidelines for IV antibiotic cover include 4-hourly penicillin or 8-hourly clindamycin. It has been recorded (personal correspondence and experience) that either mothers will 'develop an allergy' to penicillin or have heard about clindamycin therapy (it is important to check sensitivity of GBS to clindamycin).

Table 3.2 Comparison of the antibiotics benzylpenicillin and clindamycin

Drug (based on 8-hour labour)	Initial dose	Cost	Repeat doses	Cost	Total cost
Benzylpenicillin	3 g	£2.30	1.5 mg 4-hourly	£2.30	£4.60
Clindamycin	900 mg	£18.60	900 mg 8-hourly	£18.60	£37.20

The UK GBS support group advocates the use of intravenous antibiotics in labour (GBS Support 2007). Their stance on waterbirth is supportive of waterbirths, so maybe as practitioners we just need to be more creative in how we support and care for these mothers.

Plumb et al. (2007) wrote that there is no rationale for refusing mothers who have GBS a water labour/birth. There may be issues of infection control (i.e., efficient hygiene and pool cleaning) or IV antibiotic access, but these are not insurmountable. Early detection and care pathways can assist in overcoming these problems.

Care pathway suggestion for mothers with GBS infection

In some of these situations we as midwives may need to act as advocates for women, and be willing to speak out in support of mothers challenging established practices. We may also need to step outside our comfort zone and put our heads above the parapet to move things forward (Gould 2004).

The chart in Figure 3.3 and descriptions may assist midwives in assessing criteria for use of water pools. Around the world the criteria vary greatly, as I discover on professional visits. In some countries

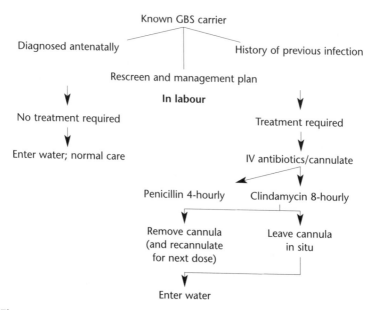

Figure 3.3 Care pathway for mother with GBS infection

mothers are supported in labouring in water/birth with GBS or if they wish a VBAC, whilst in others mothers may not even use water if they have ruptured membranes.

Criteria Risk Assessment

The following are questions for mothers to ask and midwives to answer. There are also questions midwives may wish to ask themselves. They are based on personal experience, clinical scenarios and my own literature searches.

1. Is dry land management/care transferable to water?
This is a simple question that as midwives we can review. Often care is not transferable to water: this may include any high-risk situation where continuous fetal heart rate monitoring is recommended. Another common situation is when the mother needs a cannula for receiving intravenous antibiotics. The most common reason for IV antibiotics today is with regard to group B streptococcus infection. In this situation other carers maybe involved (obstetrician/paediatrician) and there is the issue of infection control. There are ways to support mothers who wish to use water and are known to have GBS. Often this entails changing from the usual antibiotic to one called clindamycin, which is given 8-hourly rather than the traditional 4-hour regime. This may negate the issue of having a cannula in the water (those concerned with infection control worry about the mother putting her hand in the water and the dressing/cannula becoming wet). Some hospitals have restrictions on using water with GBS if the mother needs antibiotics, as the pool may be in a birth centre where IV antibiotics are not an option.

2. Does the situation/condition warrant high-risk status, based on history or evidence?
There are many studies reviewing and auditing midwifery practice, and these include aspects of high-risk mothers and babies. General audit published authors include Cluett and Bluff (2006) and Wickham (2006). However, some of the higher-risk criteria are now being challenged, one example being the use of water with GBS. Many units around the country are now allowing mothers to use water when they are known to carry GBS. The initial work was based on history but there are now audits available which support this choice. Mothers who have had a

previous Caesarean section are now starting to seek a dry land option VBAC (vaginal birth after Caesarean section), and in some enlightened units mothers are being supported to use water (sometimes for labour, not always for birth). What is important is that we review the policy for high-risk criteria, and ensure we know if it is based on history or evidence. A good example of this is scar rupture with previous Caesarean – the quoted risk is 50:10,000 (NICE 2004). This makes it very difficult for midwives, let alone mothers, to decide if this is an option that they believe is safe or realistic.

As with all aspects of using water, I suggest that you search the internet, communicate with other health professionals and balance the options for mothers.

3. Multi-professional involvement

It is important that any clinical care is designed through a multi-professional approach. There are many practitioners involved in planning care, even when booked under midwife care; we liaise with GPs and other health professionals when the need arises. As midwives we work within our professional rules and standards, which empower us to deliver safe, clinical care, summoning medical aid if needed (often only in an emergency). However, one person who can assist both midwives and mothers through challenging criteria are supervisors of midwives. This unique role in the UK provides a professional, highly skilled and senior midwife (every Trust must have supervisors) who can act as a mother's advocate in providing clear, unbiased, professional information.

In the UK there are midwives who work outside the NHS. As independent midwives they will usually be able to provide total care, including waterbirths (usually at home). All midwives within the UK work within the NMC *Midwives Rules and Standards* (2004).

4. Skills/attitudes of midwives

As midwives we have a duty of care to support mothers with a wide variety of choices. However, we also have a duty to our professional midwives' rules and standards to ensure we are 'confident and competent to undertake or develop new skills'. For some midwives, water labour/birth places a new challenge upon their skills. For many years physiological labour and birth has 'lost its way' amongst the technology of labour wards. Midwives may need to re-establish traditional skills (such as auscultation of the fetal heart with simple Dopplers), and they need to revisit criteria for using water or, indeed, physiological third stage. With waterbirth I teach midwives that they may practise a 'hands off' approach in the physical sense, partly to prevent the baby breathing under water. Much harder is the metaphorical sense: here midwives can sit, watch, learn and act when required and enjoy the energy and sense of power to be found in waterbirths.

Attitudes can be very difficult to overcome. 'Midwife' means 'with woman' and that is one beauty of water labour/birth: we can truly be with woman and experience mothers giving birth in a natural environment that they have sought out for themselves. As midwives we can share and reflect on our experiences, rationalize care and utilize others to assist in any decision-making issues. However, the issues fundamental to general attitudes, and thus often the support and number of waterbirths in a unit, is beyond the scope of this book. Other authors have written about some of these issues (Page and McCandlish 2006).

5. Mothers require informed choice not informed compliance

The 'in' expression that gets used a lot in our profession is 'informed choice', but what does this actually mean when related to waterbirth? The first question is: how many pools are available and what are the chances of a mother actually being able to get into the water? Should a mother consider a home waterbirth or can she hire a pool and bring it in? As a mother I would also want to know how many waterbirths the Trust did last year – what percentage of their normal births were water, how many women got into water and then left and why? Will there be a midwife on duty who can support you with using water or are there only a few and therefore water is available only if they happen to be on duty? We need to ensure a mother can get more information. She will want to know whether there are classes she can attend, and whether there is written information, maybe a midwife with a specialist interest who can give her realistic options and direct her to more information or support.

Nationally there are leaflets available. MIDIRS (Midwives Information and Resource Service) has informed choice leaflets and there are many websites. I believe passionately that a realistic picture should be available to women regarding informed choice rather than informed compliance (Kirkham 2009).

6. Can we offer water labour/birth and water at third stage?

When mothers think about using water it is often about waterbirth that they do the most investigation. However, there are three main areas of using water: labour, birth and third stage care. It may be possible to use water for one or all of these stages.

The best example I have is mothers who have a high body mass index (BMI). Traditionally these mothers (BMI > 30–35) have been excluded from pools. This may be due to units' reaction to CEMACH (*Confidential Enquiry into Maternal and Child Health*) or location of the pool. However, water can enhance mobility for larger mothers; it can enable them to be buoyant, the properties of water increasing weightlessness by 75 per cent. Thus larger mothers can move around more easily and benefit from the relaxation qualities of the water. The pool, of course, needs to be large enough to facilitate movement. It may still be beneficial to leave the water for delivery, but the non-intervention and labour enhancement can be very powerful both physically and emotionally.

There may be health and safety issues regarding emergency evacuation and risk assessment for these mothers, and these are discussed in Chapter 8.

7. When is the right time and place to challenge guidelines/colleagues?

As practitioners we are aware that there is a time and place to challenge both guidelines and colleagues. There may be many different avenues to discuss clinical criteria. I have mentioned the supervisor of midwives who is there to act as advocate for both mothers and midwives. The primary purpose of a supervisor is to protect the public, a role which may cause a conflict or dichotomy between two groups. However, the maternity services liaison committee has a remit to develop care and be aware of choices available to mothers; most notably, there is usually a lay chairman – actually a woman. It is recommended that she is a mother who has used the local services. Within a hospital there may also be a labour ward forum and clinical governance group. It is within these groups where as midwives we can challenge guidelines and colleagues. It should go without saying that this challenge should never be whilst a mother is actually present, nor in front of colleagues in the middle of a busy labour ward or birth centre. This causes conflict, not challenge, and will probably not be resolvable in a positive way.

8. Document and provide a clear care pathway

It is vital that, having had a discussion and gained information regarding choices about water, a clear pathway is recorded in the mother's notes. Pages 34 and 37 above show examples of care pathways for VBAC mothers and mothers with GBS infection. A similar care pathway could be adapted for mothers who fall outside a 'normality' remit or, as has occurred with the development of guidelines in some areas (see later in this chapter), a normal care pathway.

9. Audit outcomes

As part of our professional care and responsibility we are encouraged to audit practice. When waterbirths were first introduced, many of these audits were on clinical outcomes (blood loss at delivery, length of labour, perineal tears and baby Apgar scores), as the waterbirths were often on single units and the numbers were small (often less than 100). Things have changed now and there is a great deal of auditing of not only clinical outcomes, but also GBS, VBAC and mothers' decision-making experiences. There are hundreds of personal accounts of water-births from both mothers and midwives. There is a large amount of information available, which can be obtained mainly on the internet via a good search engine. Many references and websites are included within this book and within the section on websites in Chapter 11.

Guidelines for Practice

Schroeter (2004) wrote that his concerns regarding waterbirth were with regard to lack of 'controlled' RCTs (randomized control trials) – see Chapter 9. He also reports that there is no consistency in conducting a waterbirth (water temperature/depth, maternal or fetal assessments) and in reporting of adverse outcomes. Whilst in some aspects this may be true, in some countries the principles of clinical governance (see Chapter 8) are not complete, whereas in the UK these principles are maintained.

The National Institute for Health and Clinical Excellence *Intrapartum Care* guidelines (NICE 2007) identify a fundamental aspect of woman- and baby-centred care: 'Good communication is essential, supported by evidence based information, to allow women to reach informed decisions about their care.'

When waterbirths started in the UK in the mid-1980s the amount of evidence was very limited, often based on individual practitioners' experiences or small audits (Burns et al. 1993; Garland and Jones 1994; Nightingale 1994). However, by 2000 the amount of evidence from the United Kingdom and abroad has widened the information and evidence available to prospective parents and midwives.

NICE states in the guidelines that mothers should be given the opportunity to labour in water. It does not actually mention waterbirth and yet when epidurals are highlighted and documented it is clear that the risks and benefits/implications for labour are discussed. On a personal level, I would have preferred NICE to use exactly the same phrasing for water as for epidurals. I believe this is a subtle but funda-mental error on their part. There should be full and frank discussion with mothers before *any* form of analgesia is offered to a woman. Water is no different to pethidine, TENS, entonox or epidurals – there are pros and cons to all, albeit in differing ways. I would suggest that as midwives we discuss all issues of analgesia and ensure that mothers make an informed choice. There is a section called 'Coping with Pain' in the guidelines but it reads more like a checklist for midwives than a presentation of the pros and cons for us to discuss with mothers; once again, water is barely mentioned.

The NICE guidance was identified by Laurance (2007) who, as health editor of the *Independent*, wrote an article entitled 'Water birth provides the safest form of pain relief'. He wrote that waterbirths could improve the experience of maternity care for thousands of women: 'giving birth should be a normal process which ends with a spontaneous vaginal delivery where mother and baby are healthy afterwards, the guidance says. But too often, it has become a medical procedure because doctors and midwives – and mothers – become anxious about letting nature take its course.' One can only hope mothers have the opportunity to read highlights of the NICE guidelines and discuss them with their care providers.

In April 2006 the Royal College of Obstetricians and Gynaecologists (RCOG) and Royal college of Midwives (RCM) issued a joint statement regarding immersion in water during labour and birth:

Both the RCOG and RCM support labouring in water for healthy women with uncomplicated pregnancies. The evidence to support underwater birth is less clear but complications are seemingly rare. If good practice guidelines are followed in relation to infection control,

---

Box 3.1   Questions for midwives to ask of a guideline

- Is this guideline evidence informed?
- Which discipline's evidence informs it?
- Does it include midwifery evidence?
- Does it promote 'best practice'?
- Does it promote and protect the potential for physiological birth?
- Will it activate a cascade of unnecessary intervention?
- Is it appropriate for this individual woman?

Source: Banks (2009)

Table 3.3 Guidelines for practice (sample from Garland 2000a)

Midwife's clinical judgement is paramount. Establish parent's previous knowledge prior to entering water. In an emergency the mother needs to understand that she will be asked to stand/leave the pool.

Criterion for using water	Cephalic/one baby at term.
Complications	Any known or envisaged complications should have been risk assessed and a care pathway recorded (VBAC/GBS).
Induction of labour	Prostin/ARM IOL – may depend on rationale for induction, e.g., post-term.
Pregnancy induced/ essential hypertension	Evidence suggests blood pressure is lowered in hydrotherapy, so monitoring of B/P is important (Katz et al. 1990).
Ruptured membranes	24–48 hour intervention – may use water if apyrexial/CRP normal/no known pre-existing infection. Consider deep ear swab from neonate.
When to enter water	Established labour – once in labour water appears to enhance progress. Latent labour use – robust monitoring of progress of labour; no evidence needed to have a definitive cervical dilation pre-entering.
Care of mother	Basal observations pre-water. In water, check maternal temperature/pulse hourly and B/P 4-hourly. Analgesia – consider complementary therapies/inhalation (traditional therapy such as narcotics – pre-pool administration 72 hours) Ambient room temperature should be 21–22 °C; measure/record hourly. Mother should be encouraged to drink 0.5 to 1.0 litres of fluid hourly. Ensure mother voids her bladder.
Water temperature – first stage	Comfort temperature for individual mother 33–37 °C. Watch for higher temperatures as mother could become hyperthermic; record hourly.
Water temperature – second stage	Normal adult body temperature 37–37.5 °C. Record every 15 minutes. Evidence suggests that this temperature enhances labour and prevents initiation of respiration in the newborn.

Maternal position change	Use floatation aids to encourage buoyancy and mobility to reduce potential for hyperthermia/injury.
Fetal heart rate auscultation	Monitor fetal heart rate using underwater Doppler (telemetry cardiotocograph). Ensure no risk of electric shock/damage to transducer.
Care of the perineum	Traditional control of the head/guarding the perineum is not required. Reduce stimulation for first breath. Evidence suggests reduced perineal trauma as counter-pressure of water encourages slow head delivery and mother to push more steadily.
Suturing of perineum	May need to be delayed for 1 hour post-waterbirth. Perineal tissues maybe water-saturated and 'devitalized'.
Baby first breath	Non-touch technique – bring baby immediately to surface. Hypoxia may develop if baby is left underwater. There is no need to snatch baby to surface (risk of cord rupture).
Third stage management	Physiological third stage: risk assess mother – use midwives' skills. No evidence to support theory of risk of water emboli.
Estimated blood loss	Collect any clots. Record as < or > 500 ml. Assess maternal condition.
Emergency situations	Nuchal cord – never clamp and cut cord underwater. Employ skills drill for shoulder dystocia/post-partum haemorrhage. Resuscitate in close proximity. Consider lifting 'net' or hoist.
Reassessment of labour	Consider research/standard midwifery practice. Evidence suggests labour enhanced by hydrotherapy. Reassess on dry land abdominal/vaginal progress after 5 hours if delivery not imminent.
Midwifery support	Ensure midwife identifies if assistance is required prior to mother entering water.

management of cord rupture and strict adherence to eligibility criteria, these complications should be further reduced. (RCOG and RCM 2006)

When being challenged by criteria it is useful to maintain a list of mothers who may fulfil your basic criteria – one baby, head down, at term – but of course other mothers will ask to use water and as practitioners we must ensure a safe and empowering process to work with them. See the teaching quiz in Chapter 10.

Banks (2009) discusses the issue of waterbirth guidelines and how instead of supporting practice they are often interpreted as 'prescriptive care, an effective tool to rigidly control practitioners and women. The informed decision making process is negated as care is seen to be mandatory and unable to be declined or omitted ... Guidelines steer them [midwives] away from providing individualized care if they have an uncritical acceptance of them.'

Box 3.1 lists questions for midwives to think about when examining guidelines, and Table 3.3 gives a sample guideline for practice. Guidelines will be individual to each midwife's area of practice and experience, with regard to any local policies and professional codes of practice.

Reviewing Routine Care

Normality criteria may need to be challenged

This section explores some of the issues surrounding normality criteria. As a practitioner using water for many years, it has become apparent to me that we need to review what we see as 'normal'. We should remember that as far back as 1997 the RCM published *Normality in Midwifery*. Is it normal always to do an admission CTG (cardiotocograph)? What do we think happens in the community or birth centres where no CTG is available? The NICE guidelines highlight that for low-risk mothers CTGs are not required. Do we as practitioners feel confident using pinnards and fetoscopes and analysing the variability and rate as normal?

Artificial rupture of membranes (ARM)/induction of labour (IOL)

Whether we regard this as normal or not may depend on why it is being performed. Is there a clear rationale or has it become custom and practice?

Have these two interventions become so routine that we do not regard them as interventions? From my personal experience it is still routine in many countries around the world to perform an ARM at 4 cm dilation. Whilst this practice has changed dramatically in the UK, elsewhere it may still need to be challenged. It is possible to undertake an ARM under water but why would we want to interfere with the normal physiological process of labour? In a small study undertaken in 2000 at Christchurch University, Canterbury, Kent, tutors reviewed how many physiological labours and births midwifery students were being exposed to. When the interventions of induction, ARM, augmentation, epidurals, pethidine, semi-recumbent birth position, episiotomy and active third stage managements were removed, it was approximately 10 per cent of births. Is it surprising, therefore, that many midwives find it very difficult to support normal labour and birth (Garland 2000b)? What effect do all these interventions have on the physiological process?

With IOL the reason for induction needs to be clear. Is this a 'true' post-mature baby? If the mother and baby are low risk, why may they not use water? Is it because the routine is to perform a CTG every 4 hours or vaginal examinations every 2 hours? These are practices that I have come across during my travels – maybe these need to be challenged on dry land so that the opportunity is increased for these mothers to use water.

Eating and drinking in labour

Seventy per cent of women are still starved in labour, according to statistics in a recent article (Downe 2009). Whilst limiting oral nutrition in a high-risk labour is prudent (with the assumption that anaesthetists are worried about Mendelson's syndrome), for low-risk mothers there appears to be little justification for it (Curtis 1994; Davison et al. 2005; Downe 2009). However, the high-risk attitude has prevailed in many situations and mothers generally have oral nutrition withheld. For women who wish to use water this is extremely worrying, particularly with regard to fluids. As you will read in Chapter 6, I recommend a litre per hour – although most mothers drink more like 500 ml – which still maintains hydration and reduces the risk of hyperthermia and its inherent complications. So once again, as practitioners we may need to challenge established practices which have very little to do with research or practical reason, and more to do with history.

Non-directive second stage pushing

When I trained in the early 1980s I can vividly remember my community midwife assisting mothers during labour, and in particular her attitude to 'non-directive' pushing. At the time I believed this was the norm but I soon realized that this was not the case – when I attended hospital births, midwives had the 'breath holding and push three times' attitude. Having seen both options, I was very much of the opinion that mothers were able to know their own body's capability to deliver their babies.

The origin of directed pushing dates back to the eighteenth century and the physician Valsalva. This involves deep breath holding and bearing down forcibly. When a mother performs this technique major physiological changes occur (Benyon 1957; Caldeyro-Barcia 1979; Yeates et al. 1984): there is an increase in intrathoracic pressure, with a consequent drop in the venous return to the heart. This can lead to a drop in cardiac output and blood pressure (Enkin et al. 2000). There can be a consequent reduction in blood supply to the placenta and therefore less oxygen reaching the fetus. Aldrich et al. (1995), cited by Byrom and Downe (2005), discuss the effects of Valsalva-style pushing compared with the mini pushes of spontaneous pushing. They found that Valsalva pushing increases fetal heart rate abnormalities and possible interventions.

The clinical implication of this physiology is the change to the heart rate that we may experience during second stage. Enlightened midwives will often feel more confident in encouraging mothers to be instinctive with their own pushing. There is never a 100 per cent right answer to pushing – over 26 years I have seen mothers who instinctively know how to push whilst others have needed verbal encouragement. Women need to have confidence and a physiological knowledge of pushing (Lester 2008).

In waterbirths it is very unusual to undertake directive pushing; indeed, we often do not know a mother is in second stage until the vertex is visible. This often manifests itself as an apparently shorter second stage, albeit Bryom and Downe (2005) suggest that spontaneous second stage pushing leads to a longer second stage, but with no clinical relevance to fetal or maternal morbidity. The benefits of spontaneous second stage are further discussed in Chalk (2004), together with factors that are associated with spontaneous pushing:

- Spontaneous pushing is limited until the head starts to distend the pelvic floor.

- The urge to push may not commence at the onset of contraction; there may be a delay between the contraction and the urge to push.
- The amount of effort of pushing varies with each contraction.

The exact aetiology of this passive second stage in water is unknown, but certainly I believe that there is an attitude issue: the mother is more relaxed and allows normal physiology of second stage with head descent, using the lack of gravity that occurs whilst submerged in water. Whatever the reason, it is another skill that midwives often feel they need to learn when they first start waterbirths.

Relearning Traditional Skills

Diagnosing first and second stage

NICE (2007) says that in normal labour mothers may be offered vaginal examination. It does not state that all women must have a vaginal examination to assess labour, nor that mothers require 4-hourly vaginal examination – only that it should be 'offered'.

In second stage, vaginal examination is documented as being offered hourly. This is, of course, based on the care of low-risk mothers and if there is any deviation from normal then a medical practitioner is informed.

NICE also says that active second stage should be 1 hour for parous mothers and 2 hours in nulliparous mothers. What has not been identified is a passive second stage. This does not just occur with epidurals in situ; as a midwife of many years' experience I have certainly been aware of passive second stages, particularly in water but also on dry land. As a practitioner I record very clearly in my midwifery records if and when a passive second stage has occurred.

Watch, listen, learn and act/hands off

This sentiment is supported by Ponette (1999) when he wrote, 'let nature do its work as much as possible, but be alert, fast and efficient if medical action might be necessary. Only then can you reach a balance'.

Walsh (2002) wrote about how we are now starting to study the intuitive and embodied knowledge sources that may teach us much about what facilitates normal birth. This intuitive behaviour is not taught; it is learnt from our colleagues, and from mothers that we assist at birth and reflect on daily during our working lives. I also believe it is part of our life experience – who and what has influenced us in our early professional years. Midwives use (and hopefully value) other skills and senses which all play an important part in care.

I remember well my training in London with the community midwives working in a large inner-city estate. This was a council-run housing estate with a mixture of socio-economic and ethnic groups. We supported mothers at home births – not always the easiest with high parity, five floors upstairs (the lifts never seemed to be working), and with the whole family watching 'our midwife'. We sat and watched as the mothers carried on with their normal daily activities, their children around them and the labour progressing at the rate that was right for them, not dictated by a partogram (although we used one to record our observations) or action curve. In 2002 Robertson wrote that midwifery students should be exposed to home births, and as part of the registration requirement midwives should have home birth participation. Whilst I agree that home birth – and indeed waterbirth – would benefit all students, the reality is that with low home birth/waterbirth rates this maybe rather impractical.

There is a wonderful reference book by Anne Frye (2004), which is another resource about non-invasive techniques for assessing labour. Many of the tips she offers I have used in my own practice (red line developing during labour at anal margin, changes in body and verbal demeanour), but I had not heard about 'hot legs'. It has been described thus by a Mexican midwife:

> it involves noticing temperature changes on the surface of the mother's leg between the ankle and the knee. Most (but not all) women experience a temperature change in their calf when they labour. When the woman is not yet dilated, the toes and feet may be cold, but the rest of the leg is warm. As labour progresses, the line of demarcation between the cold region and the warm region moves up the leg from the ankle toward the knee. Halfway up the mother's leg is about 5 cm. When the entire calf is cold, but the knee is warm, the urge to push should follow shortly.

In water you need to wait about 15–20 minutes after leaving the water before this sign becomes reliable.

Physiological third stage

NICE (2007) suggests physiological third stage management *if requested* by low-risk women. They advise: no oxytocin, no early cord clamping, delivery by maternal effort, no pulling on cord or palpating uterus.

This has implications for midwives. How can we ensure mothers have choice with third stage unless it is discussed? What if the woman only chooses waterbirth at the end of her labour? When do we give evidence-based information? I believe that where a birthing pool is available, all mothers need to have been given information antenatally regarding third stage options. However, I do agree with the advice of no early cord clamping with physiological third stage, and that placentas are delivered attached and not clamped. A review of third stage late clamping identified that 50 per cent of the red blood cells can be lost with immediate clamping and cutting of the cord (Mercer 2001). There are issues, however, if there is nuchal cord, albeit under water. I never advocate clamping and cutting the cord under water. This will be discussed further in Chapter 7. See Box 3.2 for a summary of the issues to consider in third stage management.

It would appear that nearly 100 years ago our predecessors knew how to be patient and watchful. Fairbairn wrote in 1914 that the cardinal principle is that the attendant's attitude must be that of watchfulness only, until it can be recognized that the placenta has left the uterus and is in the vagina. If no untoward symptom occurs, necessitating active interference, nothing is done to disturb the uterus in its work of retraction and contraction; the separation and expulsion of the placenta from the uterus and the closure of the vessels in the uterine wall are allowed to take place gradually and completely, so as to minimize the dangers of postpartum haemorrhage or retention of portions of the afterbirth. As soon as there is distinct evidence that the uterus has got rid of the placenta and is firmly retracted and that these dangers are therefore no longer to be feared, efforts are made to complete delivery of the placenta.

This process may occur when a physiological undisturbed birth has occurred (see risk factors); it is in tune with the mother's body and gives her faith in her body's ability to deliver not just her baby, but also the placenta; in addition, there are benefits to the baby with physiological third stage (see Chapters 6 and 7).

This stage might be summed up by the phrase, 'It is more about what you do *not* do, rather than what you do.' Management of the third stage will be discussed in Chapter 6, 'Robust Clinical Care'.

Box 3.2 Issues for consideration in supporting physiological third stage management

Risk assessment (factors for consideration antenatally)
- Antenatal Hb
- General health and diet
- Haematological conditions – clotting disorders
- Previous labour and delivery outcomes
- Previous third stage problems – PPH/retained placenta
- Accurate maternal history – medical/surgical/obstetric

Maternal choice
- Information regarding differences between active and physiological management
- Time frames or change in management (if bleeding)
- Understanding passive third stage
- Commitment to active or physiological third stage management
- Wishing to breast feed

Midwife skills
- Knowledge and skills of risk assessment
- Clinical confidence and competence in physiological third stage
- Hands-off approach/passive third stage
- Assessing EBL (estimated blood loss)

Labour and delivery
- Nature of physiological first and second stage of labour
- Parity
- Length of labour
- Non-pharmacological analgesia (no narcotics)
- Upright/mobile first stage pre-pool use
- No augmentation – ARM (artificial rupture of membranes)
- Expected size of baby for individual mother
- No immediate cord bloods required for 'routine cord pH'
- Rhesus status and need for cord bloods
- Haematological conditions, e.g. sickle cell anaemia, requiring cord samples

Active management
1. Immediately clamp and cut cord after baby has surfaced
2. Pass baby to birth companion
3. Ask mother to leave the pool
4. Give oxytocic drug as normal on dry land
5. No delay in drug administration – suggested no longer than 10 minutes
6. Deliver placenta with controlled cord traction

Physiological
1. Leave cord attached
2. No clamping and cutting
3. Deliver placenta in or out of water
4. Lotus birth – leave placenta attached

Challenges to Practice

Challenging and supporting other professionals

As practitioners we are very aware that there is always a right time and place to challenge colleagues; the opposite is of course also true. We need to decide upon the right time, place and type of support for each other.

As a member of a caring profession, I am amazed at some of the situations I hear about. Instead of receiving support from their colleagues after a difficult situation, midwives sometimes find themselves being talked about and criticized by those same people. If a problem occurs with a delivery, we need to talk about it, reflect and learn from these experiences. When the challenge becomes a confrontational situation, midwives are likely not only back to away but possibly withdraw completely.

Fetal heart rate changes/meconium

During labour and birth we know that there may be changes to the fetal heart rate which could be either physiological or pathological. An early deceleration at 2 cm in a primigravid mother may well be managed and viewed differently from a multigravid mother at 9 cm (extremes I know) but the actions, thought processes, risk assessment etc. will empower the midwife to make a decision of physiology or pathology change.

Meconium is also a situation similar to the above fetal heart rate scenario. We assess risk factors, labour progress and other factors for deciding on physiology (term +) or pathology (fetal compromise).

This issue will be further discussed in Chapter 6.

Apgar scores

Apgar scoring has been used for many years, and although being challenged by new technology (particularly as it is not seen as a reliable predictor for long-term morbidity), it remains an important initial assessment of condition at birth. In waterbirths the most important factor is that it is truly recorded at 1 minute. The physiology of first breath in a newborn (Chapter 7) is different from that on dry land, and thus this must be allowed for with a true 1-minute Apgar. It's worth trying a trick that I use when teaching: ask your colleagues to shut their eyes, estimate a minute and when ready raise their hands. It is surprising how wide a variation you can get – 30 seconds to 2 minutes is not unusual. The bigger the group, often the bigger the gap.

Use of complementary therapies/other analgesia

Most complementary therapies sit comfortably with water (although there is disagreement between specialists regarding aromatherapy directly into the pool). Use of burners (at home), vaporizers, massage (followed by a shower before entering pool) and other forms of alternative therapies are all possible with water.

Traditional therapies are not commonly used with water. Opioids have always been the main issue of contention: when should a mother enter a pool – 3–4 hours later? The NICE (2007) guidelines say that a bath (read 'birthing pool') should not be used within 2 hours of opioids or if drowsy. Other traditional analgesics are not commonly used, although in the UK we have an inhalation analgesia called entonox (50 per cent nitrous oxide and 50 per cent oxygen), a short-acting, self-administered inhalation gas which is safe to use in water with a companion present.

Caring for your back

When birthing pools were first introduced, very few people thought about the implications for professionals' backs. However, as time has moved on it has become clear that we need to carefully identify issues around back care to reduce any potential risks and claims.

Here is a simple checklist of advice for back care for professionals:

- Attend mandatory educational sessions in conjunction with moving/handling specialists
- Risk assess any clients with raised BMIs/mobility issues
- Have practice sessions with pools, making them relevant and realistic
- Ensure all equipment is readily to hand – sonicaid/thermometers
- Have as much pool access/space as possible
- Use seating aids – stools/balls/cushions
- Practise skills drill for procedures in pool – auscultation, vaginal examination
- Practise skills drill for emergencies – shoulder dystocia, emergency evacuation
- Audit all emergencies or positioning issues.

Questions for Discussion and Reflection

- Do your guidelines reflect current practice or they based on historical evidence?
- Can you identify a mother whose condition would currently exclude her from using the pool? How would you engage with other health professionals in this situation?

4

Theories of Hydrotherapy in Labour

For many years, if you had asked midwives how water worked you would have got a shrugged shoulder response. If you were lucky you might have got a response of 'Well, it just does'! It became apparent that as midwives it was important to have more substance to the theories behind hydrotherapy, because that's what water is – a therapy.

So, back to basics. What happens when you ask a mother how she likes to relax after a day at work, getting home and everyone wanting her attention – the children, husband and pets – washing, cooking and cleaning to do? Where does she go to unwind? Many suggest that they would head to the bath to unwind. Add to this a woman with dysmenorrhoea and the rationale for using water during labour suddenly becomes far more 'natural'. What is interesting is that if you painted the same scenario to a man they would be very unlikely to offer the same way of relaxing. There does seem to be a fundamental difference between how men and women would relax. Is this important? Well I believe it could be when seeking supportive birth companions who understand the relaxing qualities of water.

Much has been written about why water assists with pain relief. I have rigorously studied evidence from both parents and clinicians and have identified four main theories behind water labour/birth.

The four theories appear to be psychological, spiritual, hormonal and physiological. All these theories have documented evidence and experiences to support the concepts explained – Simkin (1986), Gillot de Vries et al. (1987), Odent (1990), Balaskas and Gordon (1992), Jowitt (1993), Lichy and Herzberg (1993), Harper (1994) and Garland (2000a), to name but a few.

For clinical practice I will provide ideas of how to promote water and support mothers with this choice for pain relief (Benfield et al. 2007; Da Silva et al. 2007) and/or delivery. What is interesting is that we still appear to have 50 per cent of mothers who leave the water before delivery (Healthcare Commission 2008), of which a third leave because the 'quality or quantity of pain relief was not what they wanted or expected'. This phrase is important since I believe there are situations where we can encourage more mothers to stay in the water.

I also believe that expectations play a large role in the benefits of water as an analgesic. If we have faith and believe that something will assist us, it often does. If we understand the physical components (water depth and temperature) of water, it can assist us. And, finally, if we have supportive birth companions, the water is highly likely to work. It is a combination of factors that may explain why water works for one mother but not another.

Whilst all of these 'theories' have an impact on a mother's individual labour, I do not believe they are exclusive; they work together, in different amounts, at different times and in different orders. However, as a practitioner I am well aware that there are often times of variance during a labour which may impinge on each theory and these will be explored as a way of promoting water during labour. Before examining the theories, we will look at the effects of hormones in labour.

The Effects of Hormones in Labour

Adrenaline – the 'fight and flight' hormone
- Increased levels occur with fear and cold (Odent 1981)
- Increased levels can inhibit labour (Lenstrup et al. 1987)
- Adrenaline is said to trigger the fetus ejection reflex (Odent 1987)
- Studies on ewes showed that adrenaline may cause cardiovascular changes (Falconer and Powles 1982)

Catecholamines
- Normal amounts may help the fetus to withstand oxygen deprivation in labour (Simkin 1990)
- Excessive levels (through stress) may cause dysfunctional labour, decreased uterine tone, slower dilation and resulting hypoxia (Simkin 1990)
- Fetus ejection reflex occurs with increased levels (Odent 1987)
- Levels appear to increase with progressive cervical dilation (Falconer and Powles 1982)

Endorphins
- Endorphins suppress smooth muscle, relieve pain, enhance memory mechanisms, cause euphoria and regulate other hormones, such as

growth hormone, gonadotrophic releasing hormone, oestrogen and oxytocin.

- Optimal levels are reached during altered conscious state (Odent 1981)
- Normal endorphins are inhibited and suppressed by adrenaline (Milner 1988)

Oxytocin

- Optimal levels occur with altered conscious state (Odent 1981)
- Oxytocin is inhibited by the production of adrenaline, which in turn is produced by fear (Brucker 1984)

Cortisol

- High levels may suppress fetal ACTH (adrenocorticotrophic hormone) production and thereby oestriol synthesis (Maltau 1979)

I am aware that these references are old but they are seen as the original investigations of these hormonal reactions and still play an important role in understanding the role in water labour.

Circulating hormones have a profound effect on the nature of labour. Studies have been undertaken to assess the levels of oxytocin (and its use during medicalized birth) during labour. For some time it was thought that the increase in oxytocin was a linear line, but new work (not yet published) suggests that actually oxytocin rises and falls much like a wave form during labour (see Box 4.1 and Figure 4.1).

Box 4.1   Oxytocin levels

That oxytocin increases in a linear line is now being challenged by the idea of a wave form. This could have important implications for use during augmented labour. If this wave form is correct it would seem to bear out what practitioners see as the ebb and flow of labour – the natural rises and falls of physiological birth.

We are aware that there is a close relationship between stress hormones, endorphins and oxytocin. Our aim with any analgesic is to reduce the stress hormones, increase endorphins and thus oxytocin.

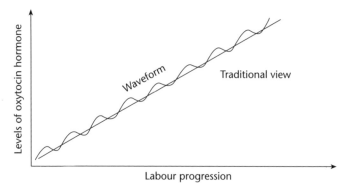

Figure 4.1   Oxytocin levels in labour

Research Relevant to Practice
A small study by Benfield et al. (2007) showed that whilst water reduced stress hormones, it also decreased levels of oxytocin and thus uterine activity. The mothers entered the water for one hour, at 3–6 cm dilated with water at 37 °C. Is water temperature or environment or birth companion involved in this process? What other factors may have played a role?
Comment: This is interesting because it appears to contraindicate other work, which shows that when stress hormones – adrenaline, noradrenaline and catecholamines –are reduced, oxytocin increases and usually causes an increase in uterine activity.

Normal Adaptive Process

The normal adaptive process (which was first described by Hans Selye, 1907–82) arises through the interplay of stress hormones (adrenaline etc.) and the release of natural analgesics (endorphins). As these are released, the hormones of labour (mainly oxytocin) are increased and labour progresses. In the situation where this normal process is impinged upon the excessive levels of stress hormones reached may actually become harmful. This may cause a shunting away of blood flow from the uterine circulation.

The process is said to assist the fetus in his preparation for extra-uterine life. With its hormonal response it

- promotes absorption of lung fluid
- protects the heart and brain
- assists the baby to maintain his body temperature.

It has been said that this normal adaptive process can cause problems if the stress hormones override labour hormones with inadequate analgesia. Many authors have written about this hormonal interplay. Below are some of those authors and an outline of the effects of hormones on labour.

Simkin (1986)

A certain amount of stress is harmless to mother and baby in labour. Excessive stress increases maternal catecholamines and can be related to dysfunctional labour (decreasing uterine tone, slowing dilation)/fetal or neonatal distress. Adaptive response, i.e. stress in normal labour, is harmless and of benefit to a healthy baby,

Lichy and Herzberg (1993)

Stress hormones increase catecholamines with fear; the primitive survival mechanism slows or stops labour. Water reduces fear and pain; it aids mobility, comfort and familiarity. Endorphins, our natural painkillers, increase a sense of wellbeing and have an amnesic effect.

The authors found that after they are 4–5 cm dilated mothers are more relaxed, so produce more endorphins. This biofeedback can be interrupted by people or surroundings and cause a disruption to this process.

Jowitt (1993)

Jowitt wrote about beta endorphins, which have both physiological and psychological effects. They suppress smooth muscle, relieve pain and produce a euphoria-like sensation (similar to pethidine and opiates). In labour they are released when a woman is relaxed; however, when she becomes stressed levels rise and can have a profound effect on oxytocin production.

There is a very fine interplay between all hormones and it is important to maintain this balance in labour. We need to support women in relaxing (thus allowing beta endorphins to rise) and reduce stress, which can increase beta endorphins to a level so high they can actually reduce the amount of oxytocin produced and thus slow the labour.

Theory 1: Psychological

Environment, in this situation, is about the room where labour is to take place. Mothers often describe in great detail the pictures and décor, which may have been designed by midwives or as a community project. The environment certainly needs to be relaxing, and so consideration needs to be given to lighting, heating, ventilation, music and distractions. This is only part of the story, but these elements all have a part to play in supporting the woman.

The role of birth companions has been discussed for many years, particularly the issue of the place of a man at birth. In my career we appear to have changed our minds about whether they should or should not be present. After nearly 30 years, the jury is still out, as they say. Certainly, having a supportive birth companion who can communicate the mother's wishes (with or without a written birth plan) is invaluable. They would have discussed choices and wishes and would have thought about this birth experience; I have seen both sides of the coin at home/hospital, in water and on dry land. Birth companions, whether male or female, family or friends, professional doulas or not, are invaluable if they are committed and supportive, do not exude anxiety and are willing to be involved. Howsen (2009) has written widely about the father's role at birth: 'the transition to fatherhood is one of the most significant and challenging experiences a man will ever face ... we need to provide appropriate educational, physical and emotional support for "father love"'.

Gillot de Vries et al. (1987) wrote that women who used water felt it was a positive experience and expressed satisfaction with the water (200 women). Women appear to enjoy a better level of consciousness during delivery, felt secure in their environment and with their birth partners, and established early mother–child interaction.

Theory 2: Spiritual

The deep relaxation that mothers experience can be described as physiological and not pathological (drug-induced regression). A mother may describe feeling 'zoned out' or spaced out, and as practitioners we may need to remind ourselves that she has not had a narcotic analgesia (pethidine or Demoral). However, the benefit of this type of regression is that if you suddenly ask a woman to stand up, she will be immediately alert. Mothers often describe this zoning out in similar terms to hypnobirthing: they are aware that we are present, quietly in the background but not intruding. This peaceful regression is often described as part of the 'aah' effect.

Many authors have written about this spiritual zoning out. Ray (1986) describes a spiritual level of regression in water. Odent (1990) explores some of the lateral concepts of water labour/birth and why women may choose this option. Wielder (1999) says, 'The less involved and more natural the birthing process, the more rewarding are the results', reminding us that water is a healer: we are nourished in it, born into it, and return there to relax and exercise; we are made up of water, and drink it to survive.

Theory 3: Hormonal

From the theories point of view, I believe that the hormonal feedback is the most powerful effect that water can enhance during labour. Odent (1990) wrote that water reduces stress hormones, reduces gravity, and encourages sensory stimulation and relaxation.

Figure 4.2 aims to show simplistically the biohormonal feedback between adrenaline, noradrenaline, catecholamines (the so-called stress

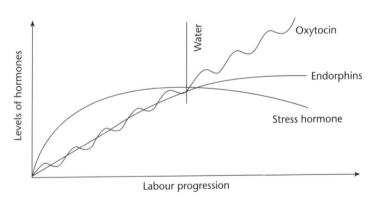

Figure 4.2   Biohormonal feedback

hormones), endorphins (natural painkillers) and oxytocin (contraction hormone).

Theory 4: Physiological

The physiological benefits of water include (a) buoyancy, which causes joint decompression; (b) reduction in viscosity of muscles; (c) enhancement of sensory stimulation and increased circulation; (d) increased lymphatic and venous flow, which helps to clear waste products. Miller and Magill-Cuerden (2006) have stressed the importance of having access to water, and Miller writes in the NCT *Creating a Better Birth Environment* survey (Newburn and Singh 2003) that the majority of women said that access to a bath or birthing pool enhanced labour.

Water has hydrothermic and hydrokinetic properties. The hydrothermic effect arises from water being a conductor of heat, which helps to relieve muscle spasm and thus pain. The warm water induces local vasodilation, increase in nerve conduction velocity and muscle relaxation. The warmth also provides comfort for the mother. The hydrokinetic effect is the abolition of gravity. This gives mothers buoyancy and allows them to float; the displaced water equals the weight loss that the mother will experience (Skinner et al. 1986; Edlich et al. 1987; Mackay 2001). Both these two properties are thought to combine in assisting relaxation and reducing anxiety.

Hydrostatic properties occur when a body is submerged and at rest (is labour at rest?). The hydrostatic pressure is the same in all directions and equally distributed at any given depth beneath the surface of the water. So instead of the full force of gravity and localized pressure of the bed beneath her, a mother who labours in warm water receives equal pressure, and support on all body surfaces submerged beneath the water. Edlich et al. (1987) highlighted the importance of the water being deep enough to allow this submerged position. Often described as the 'aah' feeling when a mother first gets into the water, this sensation has been well documented by mothers and caregivers alike.

Richmond (2003) noted that B/P (blood pressure) was lower once a mother entered the water. Whilst initially thought to be of benefit (Doniec-Ulman et al. 1987), caution was advised by Zimmerman in 1993, who stated that whilst the B/P reduction may be useful for mothers with primary hypertension (I have used water immersion for mothers with essential hypertension and pregnancy-induced hypertension), there maybe a theoretical risk of decreased placental transfusion.

It may be that ensuring robust measurement of maternal B/P pre- and post-water immersion and fetal heart rate auscultation could give early warning of problems. Although I have never heard of a mother with essential hypertension or pregnancy-induced hypertension experiencing any problems, it may be prudent for these women to have their blood pressure checked every 15 minutes for the first hour to ensure a normotensive blood pressure and no hypotensive events that could compromise mother or baby. It is also essential that we differentiate between pregnancy-induced hypertension and pre-eclampsia (using blood results, fetal growth scans, Doppler studies).

Water may also act as a distraction and work in a way similar to the gate control theory (similar to TENs) with release of endorphins, endogenous hormones and subsequent pain control (Brucker 1984).

The effect of immersion in water is a positive pressure on the body, producing significant diuresis and natriuresis (the excretion of greater amounts of sodium in the urine). There may also be an antidiuretic hormone effect or even a shift in tissue fluid into the blood. The amount of literature about this with regard to adults is very limited and almost nothing is written from a pregnant mother's perspective.

Newburgh (1968) wrote about circulating adrenaline causing modifications in the circulation, which favours blood supply to active muscle, liberation of glucose from glycogen and increased heat production.

Enhancing the Qualities of Water

The 'aah' effect is not usually apparent until the mother feels physically and psychologically relaxed. It appears to take about an hour for the theories of water to take effect. So it is important to think about these theories if water does not appear to be enhancing labour and providing analgesia. The following simple guide may assist when a mother says the water is not working and she wishes to leave. Think about the various elements.

Psychological

Environment: room relaxing not overwhelming; calming colours
Room: light – over-pool lights, twinkle lights, tea lights, torches;
　　heat – fans to cool; check windows for draughts
Caregivers: watch for negativity; be confident and competent; ensure support from co-ordinators/colleagues

Birth companions: are they really committed?; female or male?; non-fussy, supportive?

Spiritual

Ensure minimal noise; relaxed and supportive environment for both mother and caregiver/partner; balanced light and ambient temperature; minimal distractions.

Hormonal

Hormones reduce stress, helping mother to relax and 'zone out'.

Physiological

Consider water depth and temperature; mobility; supply adequate floatation aids.

When I introduced these theories in early 1990 to the midwives, we re-audited a year later and reduced by half the number of mothers who left the water due to analgesia effectiveness.

Questions for Discussion and Reflection

- Reflect on these theories when caring for a mother in the water to enhance the experience of analgesia.
- Could you utilize these theories in other care settings?

5

Engaging with Parents

What can we do, as midwives, to engage with parents and promote water labour/birth as an option?

It sounds logical to say that we should have effective communication systems with mothers, but studies have shown (Alexander et al. 1993) that the information given and received by different client groups varies greatly depending on social, ethnic and cultural backgrounds. Communication with mothers may occur through various avenues – verbal, written or electronic. Whichever is used, it is vital that it is clear, up-to-date and unbiased and that it offers mothers informed choice regarding waterbirth. The challenge for health professionals is to ensure this is done for all parents regardless of background and of our own possible positive or negative opinions.

I will explore individual and group parent education classes, aquanatal swimming, individual risk assessment, clinical governance and using the media. This chapter will also identify leaflets, websites and other literature suitable for prospective parents.

Choosing a Pool

There are many helpful websites and articles that can assist parents in choosing the right pool for them. There are several issues to consider.

At home: Is your floor strong enough? I have known of waterbirths occurring in top-floor flats, eighteenth-century cottages, modern and old terrace houses, mostly on the ground floor. Some parts of a floor maybe stronger than others; if you live in a Victorian terrace you may have a cellar no longer used but still present, which means a weaker floor. Pool manufacturers say that even the heaviest pool, when full, weighs no more that 10–12 adults, so that gives you a guide.

Pools vary in their dimensions, depths and materials of construction. I always suggest that, especially at home, parents mark out the dimensions on the floor and measure the space available. It is important that the depth, width and weight are all suitable. With so many pools available parents have a wide choice to achieve the optimum size for them, particularly if a birth companion is planning to get into the pool. The weight of the pool should be worked out and the setting considered in relation to what I have said above about floor strength. I have never heard of pool structural problems except those seen in TV programmes (*William and Mary*, UK, mid-2000 and *Men Behaving Badly*, UK, 1990s) but it makes sense to check.

In hospital: In hospitals I usually suggest that where possible go for the largest pool you can afford. Ask colleagues whether, if they were to spend their money again, they would buy this particular pool; if they say 'no', ask why not. A large pool, with clever use of floatation aids, can be made to seem smaller; but of course it is impossible to make a small one bigger once installed.

Remember that 75 per cent of the mother's body weight will alter as she becomes buoyant, allowing her to move with ease, change position and benefit from the relaxation the water offers. So the pool must be the right size for the mother. If she is not hiring and plans to use a pool in a hospital or birth centre setting, there are certain things we as midwives can do to ensure the appropriate size of pool.

A reported injury in Ahmed and Patel (2005) highlighted the importance of a woman regularly changing her position in the water. The mother was on 'all fours', knees flexed and wide hips. The birth lasted approximately 6 hours. On leaving the pool the mother noted tingling and numbness in the antero-lateral aspect of her right leg. She also experienced some foot drop. It is not documented how often she changed position, nor the type of pool, nor how long she was actually in the pool. Whilst only one or two such incidents have been reported, it is important to ensure the mother alters position regularly. We should remember that such leg/back problems do occasionally occur after an epidural – although they may not be publicized.

Parent Information

Classes

In some areas of midwifery, the response to local needs has been the introduction of specific antenatal waterbirth classes. It is important to ensure that mothers have access to evidence-based information to make an informed choice, and to be realistic and practical with the information given. I have found that being honest saves parents being disappointed on the day: they need to understand that there may be a limited number of midwives who can support waterbirths, or only one pool available, or certain exclusion criteria.

The classes may be separate from routine classes and specific to your client group. They may be specific to age, ethnic background or religious group. Particular groups may be targeted for particular reasons, such as non-attendance at appointments or requirements about dignity in the pool (I have known of mothers wearing burkas in the water in order to overcome religious/cultural concerns) or about water being 'unclean' because it has body fluids within it.

The content of the classes will vary but in the classes I run I cover the following:

- Why water? – from the mother's point of view
- When to get in/out of water
- Caring for you and your baby
- Partner's role
- Short film
- Tour of pool room

Leaflets

Many midwives decide that they want separate leaflets about waterbirth; others may decide to combine the waterbirth information with other forms of natural analgesia (e.g., TENS, birthing balls, aromatherapy). The decision needs to be made based on the client group, finances and types of other leaflets available. One issue is paramount: the quality of the leaflet must be similar to others available (I have seen a unit with glossy, mass-produced, colour epidural leaflets whilst the waterbirth one was a photocopy of a photocopy of a photocopy – hardly presenting a balanced view).

Websites

There are hundreds of websites which mothers may access. Type 'waterbirth' in the search engine of your computer and you will have an array of sites, mothers, companies and professionals. Before I recommend any site I always review it myself to ensure it is relevant to the mothers I work with. Many are international and do not always transfer to your own country.

Research Relevant to Practice

Richmond (2003) took a sample of 240 waterbirths from a total of 482 waterbirths in a unit in south-east England. 78% thought it seemed natural, 78% thought it would be less painful, 72% thought it would be gentle for baby, 50% wanted drug-free labour, 37% thought there would be less tearing, 27% had it recommended, and 24% wanted reduced interference.

Comment: The majority – 64% – heard about waterbirth via the media and only 17% via the midwife, which suggests that midwives have more to do in terms of publicity.

Aquanatal Preparation

As early as the eighteenth century, books were being printed in London (Baylies 1757; Falconer 1770) extolling the virtues and benefits of water for all kinds of conditions, including pregnancy and labour. Maybe there is a long history of using water and the stories told of historical water labours and births may actually have some substance. Whilst I do not advocate that antenatal use of water should be a prerequisite for underwater birth, I do believe that as an adjunct it is very beneficial.

Swimming has long been known as an enjoyable and strong relaxant. It is something that every member of the family can enjoy and it bestows positive health benefits. Water can be used by even the most compromised individual, and for expectant mothers it can, therefore, be a most beneficial form of exercise and relaxation. It can also be undertaken and extended into the postnatal period by both mother and baby. Aquavie, a company that promotes antenatal swimming, state on their website that good swimming techniques that provide relaxation and exercise should not include breaststroke, since it could cause severe pain in the mother's back or neck, due to poor spinal alignment. It is therefore prudent that mothers ensure, before undertaking an aquanatal class, that it is run by a professional, qualified antenatal water educator.

As health professionals we aim to promote physical and mental well-being for women during their pregnancy. They are encouraged not to smoke or drink, and to attend antenatal care and classes in order to prepare themselves for labour and birth. Some people liken labour to running a marathon. No athlete would enter a race without adequate preparation, and yet many mothers appear to do little physical preparation. As midwives we have contact with mothers for 9 months, which allows us to plan for the labour and birth ahead.

Research Relevant to Practice

Katz et al. (1988) reviewed the fetal–maternal homeostasis when exercising in water. There was no reported elevation in rectal temperature and the plasma volume levels remained stable. Maternal temperature and heart rates were unchanged and ultrasound scans showed all fetuses were in an active state during immersion.

Finding an organized class

Throughout the UK there are many organized classes run by qualified and organized professionals. Many have undertaken an aquanatal course, which assists in not just the content – physical exercise and relaxation – but also the organization of a class.

Midwives who wish to start classes should ensure they are appropriately qualified, have reviewed their own professional code of practice (acquiring new skills) and have some degree of business acumen (accounts/costings/overheads). A female life saver should be available and there should be at least two midwives at each class, one to teach and one to be in the pool. It is advisable not to wear any distracting jewellery, and access to music seems to help – 'golden oldies' seem to work well with pool acoustics! Box 5.1 lists important elements to consider.

Benefits of aquanatal classes include psychological and physiological preparation. This has been demonstrated to the full in Ostend, Belgium, at the New Aquatic Birth Centre. The antenatal experience there includes swimming, exercising and relaxing in a seawater swimming pool. Parents then return with their newborns for a weekly swim.

This preparation is a comprehensive education programme – Aquarius – which uses physical and mental preparation. Water exercises and relaxation are complemented with a practical course in the symbolic meaning of water, looking at benefits and also fears of water. The water exercises allow mothers to free themselves from the fear of water, to develop trust and confidence in themselves. They encourage mothers to become aware of their breathing, developing rhythmic and

---

Box 5.1   Administration of aquafit classes

Pool – graduated depths; access via stairs not a ladder
Deeper water allows for greater water pressure resistance
Shallow water will encourage non-swimmers to participate
Aim for exclusive use – especially for mothers from ethnic minorities

Pool safety – check fire exits/drills
Mobility access
Floatation aids

Water temperature – 28–30 °C reduces tension and relaxes muscles
If too cool, women may get muscle cramps
If too hot, women may feel dizzy and lethargic

Changing room – privacy; individual cubicles
Space to wheel in prams – if postnatal class is run

Cost and advertising – hire whole pool/specific sessions
Advertise local newspapers/consumer groups
Speak on local radio/TV

Professional indemnity – check with your professional organization
Consider conflict of interests with employer

Mothers' preparation – questionnaire to mothers concerning general health
Discuss current pregnancy issues
Allow time to unwind after class – usually 20 mins
Source: Halksworth (1994), Cain (1992), Baddeley (1999)

---

deep breathing. Water relaxation is based on floating techniques similar to watsu. The theoretical course allows mothers to gain an insight into fetal life and the structure and purpose of the course. Postnatal water classes for mothers and babies are introduced and the programme concludes with a visit to the aquatic maternity centre in Ostend. Details can be found in Chapter 11 in the section on DVDs.

Aqualight, published by Birthlight, is a series of exercises enabling women to get the best out of a birthing pool before, during and after birth. The photographs and short descriptions enable mothers to use water to stretch muscles and widen pelvic diameters during pregnancy. For labour and delivery the pool is shown with models in various positions, including kneeling. The booklet also shows the pool being used for the newborn's first floating experience. See details in the section on websites in Chapter 11.

Box 5.2   Benefits of aquanatal classes

Physiological benefits
Fitness levels maintained during pregnancy
Exercise not based on previous exercise history
Assists in controlling weight
Reduces muscle tension such as backache
Improves posture and mobility
Reduces varicose veins and swollen ankles
May reduce blood pressure
Reduces stress hormones

Psychological benefits
Women's morale and self-esteem improved
Improves mobility – 75% weight reduction during immersion
Social event for mothers
Water is environmentally friendly

Source: Reid-Campion (1990)

The benefits of aquanatal classes are shown in Box 5.2. Many mothers, having experienced antenatal swimming, wish to continue with this postnatally. Exercises postnatally concentrate on thighs and waistlines. Ideally we like mothers to exercise for life but in today's economic situation we are glad if we see them with us for 3 months. I usually advise mothers to wait for their 6-week postnatal examination before recommencing, and for those who have had a Caesarean section to get a medical opinion. A simple rule of thumb is that by 6 weeks bleeding will have stopped and sutures will have healed.

Many other classes run alongside antenatal classes. Local classes start with postnatal and finish with antenatal mothers, which gives mothers a chance to dry themselves, settle their babies and hopefully meet pregnant mothers over a cup of coffee.

Many colleagues offer water to a wider group of mothers, such as mother and baby classes. I experienced this opportunity in Israel during a professional visit in 2008. These classes offer parents the chance to develop newborn development and interaction, and mothers and babies appear to really enjoy this activity. Freud wrote, 'Never underestimate the importance of play.'

Some practitioners find this water activity gives other benefits to newborns; these can be heard or read about from the practitioners in Ostend, Belgium (see Chapter 11).

The disadvantages of aquafit need also to be considered, and these are shown in Box 5.3.

> **Box 5.3   Disadvantages and contraindications of aquafit**
>
> • Substantial initial start-up costs
> • Problems in finding a suitable pool
> • Training of midwives – cost and time
> • Pool must be kept clean at all times – MRSA does not grow in water
> • Slips/injuries – very rare if precautions taken

Specific clients

If you encounter mothers who do not fulfil your client criteria for using the pool you may need to involve your manager or, in the UK, supervisor of midwives. I know of several units in the UK which ask a mother to sign to say that she wishes to use water for labour/delivery and has seen and read the midwifery guideline for waterbirth. I would fully support providing client information, discussing it in parent education classes and giving it to the woman to read with her partner. Whether it is legally binding to sign that they have accepted a guideline that cannot cover all risk assessment as labour progresses is uncertain; it could be interesting if challenged in law. Do these units believe that this would stand up in court if there was any litigation; and what happens if the mother says she signed it so she had a chance to use water and was put under extreme duress?

Some clients may benefit from extra professional support (those with mobility problems, VBAC or previous neonatal issues) but they should all be individually assessed. If we do not aim to provide a safe and realistic care pathway (see Chapter 3 for examples) then these mothers may opt out of the health systems and free birth. In one large teaching hospital in London they have an 'out of criteria clinic', a unique system to ensure mothers can access up-to-date information, evidence and options for their choices of care.

Publicity

Local newspapers and radio will often do articles on waterbirths; they appear to like anything to do with mothers and babies. Whether you are launching a new service or developing an old one, starting up classes or buying a new pool, utilize the local media services. If you are a person who likes to write or speak, find the person who is writing the article and offer to assist them with being the contact, or photo finder (there are lots on the internet). You might be someone who is good with statistics and can add those to the article. If possible, write something for local consumer magazines (ideally with one of the local waterbirth mothers) and remember that 'pictures say a thousand words'; subtle pictures can easily be edited for local papers.

And finally ...

The Darzi Report (DoH 2008) raises the issue that for the first time it will be expected that information about the quality of care will be measured and published by UK hospitals. It will no longer be just about numbers, a point that is relevant to maternity care, which is often to do with quality not just outcome. Mothers may have a vaginal birth but with syntocinon, an epidural or episiotomy. They should now have the opportunity to have access to data about 'quality' issues and not just percentages.

Questions for Discussion and Reflection

- How do you interact with mothers to ensure they have access to information and support regarding waterbirth?
- Is waterbirth included in parent education classes/leaflets?

6

Robust Clinical Care

Paramount to a safe service are midwives who feel confident and competent in offering water labour/birth. This chapter will discuss the latest clinical guidelines from the RCOG and RCM (2006). I will identify safe clinical parameters for care, including water temperature, maternal and fetal observations and 'What if ... ?' scenarios when things do not go to plan. This will also include emergency evacuation from the pool.

Family-centred Care

Many women seem to choose water as a way of bringing the whole family together. I have witnessed this at home, in birth centres and in hospitals – often with interesting results. In an American birth centre (Goshen, Indiana) I was privileged to witness a family waterbirth: both sets of grandparents (who stayed in the family room with the three other children) and the partner who got involved by getting into the pool (Figure 6.1 shows a couple in the pool together). When it became apparent that the woman was about to deliver, she asked if the children could come in; they had been well prepared and had disposable cameras with them to record the event. The children accepted what was happening and showed no fear or concern; they appeared to feel this was normal. As at a home birth, where I advocate that there is a birth companion for the children, these girls were lucky they had grandparents and an English midwife! Children are often far more resilient about birth than we give them credit for.

Other members of the family should not be forgotten: animals seem to have a real interest in birthing pools, often just the right height for 'lapping bowls' for larger dogs, and cats like to walk around the edge of pools. Just remember that if it's an inflatable pool and you frighten the cat, you may end up with a burst edge, and several hundred litres of water on the floor!

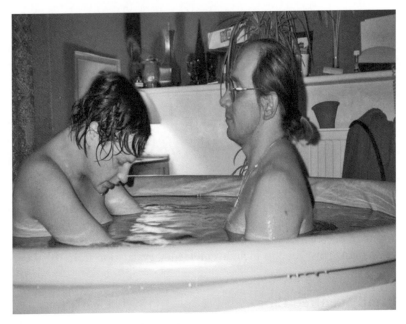

Figure 6.1 Partner in the pool

On a serious note, it is important to be conscious about health and safety with young children who may find the pool very interesting – be careful of pool depth and temperature of water, both potentially serious problems and ones I always discuss with parents who are thinking of buying or hiring a pool for home use.

Maternal and Newborn Care

Maternal observations

Before a mother enters the water I recommend basic basal observations are performed. If these basic observations are taken as suggested below, a change can be rationalized with regard to physiological change (water too hot) or pathological (infection).

I recommend that the following observations are made:

- *Temperature*: hourly once in pool to reduce risk of hyperthermia
- *Pulse*: every 15 to 30 minutes
- *Blood pressure*: 1–4 hourly, depending on current dry land care.

Harper (2005) cites Dr Serge Weisel in stating that there can be a decrease in heart rate and blood pressure of 10–15 mmHg diastolic. Weston et al. (1987) also write that there can be a reduction of blood pressure when in water: 9 mmHg at 33 °C, 18 mmHg at 37 °C and 30 mmHg at 39 °C. For mothers with pregnancy-induced hypertension or essential hypertension, this could be a useful reduction, as long as it is combined with careful observation of maternal and fetal wellbeing. However, many mothers with raised blood pressure are excluded from using water.

Analgesia in water

As a rule of thumb, most traditional forms of analgesia (narcotics/epidural) do not go well with water, whilst most complementary therapies are suitable for use with water.

Traditional analgesia

- Entonox: suitable in water but do not leave the mother unattended.
- Narcotics: not usually advised whilst the mother is in the pool. If given before pool entry, check that she is not drowsy and that the fetal heart is audible within normal variability. Life span of the drug (usually 2–4 hours) needs to be considered (NICE 2007).
- Epidurals: not suitable in water, but I have heard of a unit in South America where spinal analgesia is inserted and the woman then lowered into the water.

Complementary therapies

All forms of therapy are suitable with water – reflexology, herbals, acupuncture, homeopathy. The only therapy that divides opinion is aromatherapy with regard to direct use into water. Burns and Kitzinger (2000) and Tiran and Mack (2000) – both well-known midwife authors – do not agree. Its use will depend on your skills and knowledge of aromatherapy, local guidelines and national policies. The difference of opinion is with regard to the danger of absorption of the oil through the mucus membranes of the baby's eyes if he/she is delivered under water. It is not advised that pure aromatherapy oils are used on newborns.

It is difficult to decide on whether to use aromatherapy when two specialists do not agree. I do use aromatherapy but only with massage or inhalation. If the mother then wishes to use water I advise her to have a shower before entering the pool. I would not add aromatherapy oils directly into the water.

Fetal heart rate

Monitoring of the fetal heart should be in line with dry land management (NICE 2007): every 15 minutes after a contraction once in established labour, and every 5 minutes after a contraction in second stage. Which piece of equipment is used may be based on what the mother wishes, familiarity of equipment and practicalities. Under water the easiest is an underwater Doppler, or a fetoscope/pinards stethoscope if the mother does not wish for any electronic equipment (take care with your back); and if high risk, a telemetry CTG.

Mobility/floatation aids

Harper (2002) writes that body weight distribution is 75 per cent less in water that is up to breast level. We can facilitate this by ensuring we have floatation aids available which can be easily cleaned for multiple use. The simplest are swimming aids and bath pillows, the more fun and colourful the better. In some places mothers have to bring their own because the infection control staff do not believe they can be adequately cleaned, although I have never heard of any cross-infection situations if strict cleaning protocols are followed.

Fluids

Mothers need to drink a large amount of fluid to remain hydrated. I usually have a visual guide for a mother and her partner to remind them it should be about a litre an hour. Human nature, however, tends to reduce this to 500 ml, which is probably the minimum she needs to remain hydrated.

Women will always worry about how they void. There are several options: get out, stand up with a small container between the legs or void in the pool. If a woman expresses concern about this I remind her that it is her urine, it is sterile, it is concentrated and then diluted in 100 gallons or more of water. She should be reminded that the midwife needs to know she has voided so it can be documented (basic bladder care). The biggest problem is often psychological – mothers do not always like the idea of voiding in water. If that is the case, it is best to leave the water and go to the toilet.

Mirrors

A mirror can be a useful aid in water: for midwives who feel that they need to be able to see what is happening, and for mothers to encourage them with the descent of the baby. Many mirrors have a problem with cleaning and therefore multiple use, and this can be a problem. In the UK an independent midwife has developed a mirror specifically designed for use with water and has no problem with the cleaning of it. However, the other issue with mirrors is about our need to visualize and maybe 'control' the delivery. Support is fine but control is more fundamental to our attitudes.

Sieves/disposable containers

Any body material in the pool should be removed. On a general level, most women and midwives will not find it pleasant to have body materials in the pool. On a serious level, see the 'What if ... ?' section towards the end of this chapter concerning an adverse outcome with faecal contamination. I also mention this as a reminder that if there is severe faecal contamination in the second stage, this is very unusual and may indicate that the mother is not fully dilated. It is very unusual (unlike dry land) that the mother pushes and passes a bowel movement. One reason is physiological – mothers have a passive second stage and therefore would not normally have a bowel motion in water. Physiologically, the second stage is often very passive.

Flashlights/torch

Some of the expensive pools have built-in lighting; otherwise, midwives may purchase flashlights (even underwater diving lights) to assist in seeing the birth. Mothers often wish the room to be dark; however, midwives find it hard not to be able either to see the birth or write their records. Another alternative is a cycle head-lamp which can be worn during birth and record writing – it may look strange but it works well.

Water temperature

For many years the issue of delivery water temperature has been based on the assumption that the newborn should be delivered into water at normal adult body temperature. Indeed, I have personally taught this and used it in extensive clinical practice since my first waterbirth in 1987.

In 2004 Anderson highlighted some of the issues raised by practitioners regarding birth delivery water temperature. In this article she cites other authors who are aware of waterbirths occurring in Russia, Japan (ocean births) and Germany (pool births), where water temperature is not considered such an issue. Indeed Geissbuehler et al. (2002), in a small study carried out in Switzerland, allowed mothers to fill birthing pools to their own choice of temperature. The range was intriguing: from 33 °C to 38.2 °C. The mother's temperature remained normal; the authors believe mammals are able to maintain their temperatures at a homeostasis thermal level. Anderson (2004) believes that the thermometers should be thrown out and that we should acknowledge that labouring mothers are able to control their temperatures through normal mammalian capacity for thermostasis. These sentiments are supported by Harper (2002), writing about a variety of waterbirths occurring around the world in 'non-temperature measured water'.

Cornelia Enning (2007) discusses water as a medium for undisturbed physiological birth. She writes that water has been known as a healer since the sixteenth century. Unlike most other practitioners (except those delivering in the ocean), she uses much lower water temperatures for labour, believing that the cooler the water the more buoyant the mother. Delivery temperature is also much cooler than other practitioners use. Most practitioners appear to agree that for labour a standard of 'comfort' temperature is satisfactory. However, very hot (37+ °C/98 °F) or very cool (34 °C/92 °F) temperatures may slow a labour down as the body diverts its energies to keep the woman cool or warm. I have experienced this phenomenon myself: when the water was very cool, at 34 °C, the mother's labour slowed down, with contractions only coming every 3–5 minutes. Subtly, the water was warmed up to 36+ °C and then the nature of the labour changed – contractions became more frequent and stronger. Of course, it is vital to ensure water, room and maternal temperature are monitored and this is discussed further on in this chapter. Remember that the higher temperatures of water need to be carefully monitored and the implications of maternal hyperthermia fully understood (maternal pyrexia and tachycardia leading to fetal hyperthermia and possible cerebral compromise). See Chapter 7 and Appendix 2.

The biggest controversy is regarding water temperature at birth and this is discussed in Chapter 3.

Clarity of water

The water generally remains very clear during labour and birth, although during the third stage (if the mother chooses to stay in the water for placental delivery) there may well be a certain amount of loss of water clarity. If the water were not clear, we would not get the beautiful clear photography we see on DVD and still photographs. In fact, it is this clarity that assists practitioners in highlighting when a mother may be bleeding, some time before haemodynamic changes occur or the mother says she is feeling faint. Postpartum haemorrhage will be discussed later in this chapter.

I have seen inventive ways of ensuring clarity of the pool. In portable pools that have clear liners, midwives get mothers to write words of affirmation or enlarged photos of their baby scan, which are placed on the bottom of the pool. As this is the deepest part of the pool, if any contamination or bleeding occurs you lose sight of the words/photo. This will then indicate that the mother is possibly having a problem, and before she feels unwell and cannot stand up, you can ask her to leave the water.

I have experienced only two situations of body fluid contamination which have required me to ask mothers to leave the water so that we can empty the pool, and clean and fill it with fresh water. Both mothers had taken bottles of castor oil the night before. One mother only showed that she was in second stage when she was sick into the water as she passively pushed! This woman was being induced; she was finding the induction process very painful with prostaglandin pessaries, and was asking for an epidural at 2 cm. However, as we walked over to the labour ward I saw the anaesthetist heading towards theatre, so I realized that no epidural would be available for some time. Mainly as a stopgap, I offered the pool to the mother, who initially was not keen (she did not want a narcotic either). Her husband was also finding the situation distressing, so once this mother was settled into the water I sent him away to have breakfast. We settled into the pool room, the lights low and music quietly playing in the background. She appeared to achieve the 'aah' effect quickly (see Chapter 4). When her husband returned, he was surprised at how relaxed she was, so I left the room to give the couple some time to themselves, returning every 15 minutes to auscultate the fetal heart. After about an hour the husband called me back and said she had been sick in the water. As we were deciding what to do, I glanced down and saw the baby's head just sitting there. She delivered her own baby and brought it to the surface with no obvious ill effects of the water contamination.

A word of caution, however, should be sounded: we must ensure that the water does not become over-contaminated. In the CEMACH report of 2000–1, *Why Mothers Die*, there was a report of the death of a mother following a waterbirth where the water was contaminated with faecal matter. She became unwell and developed a temperature of 40 °C, with pain and infection in her buttock and leg. She continued to be overwhelmed by sepsis and died despite intensive medical and surgical treatment. The exact aetiology of this situation is of course not clear, but it must certainly highlight the importance of the water being kept clear.

Assessing Labour

When I started practising waterbirth in 1987 there was a general feeling amongst colleagues that women should not enter the water until 4–5 cm dilated. This became an arbitrary figure and as such a starting point for entering the water. The wisdom of the day seemed to be that if women entered the water too early the labour would slow or stop. But we need to ask: too early for whom – the mother, the midwife or even the unit?

Here is an example from my own practice. I cared for a woman who was being induced for pelvic girdle pain. All parameters were normal but she was finding the prostin contractions extremely painful. As we had made a commitment to deliver this mother, it was felt that although 'she was rather early for an epidural' (to quote the anaesthetist), we could go to the labour ward and have one performed. When we got to the ward I explained the options for analgesia. I was very careful to introduce water as 'hydrotherapy analgesia' and not just water. This woman's partner was very resistant: he said she had already been in a bath – but not a bath like the one on the labour ward, which I duly showed to both parents. I stayed with the mother whilst we added water to the right temperature for her, lowered the lights, played some relaxing music and chatted. She floated on the floatation aids and was actually humming to the music. Her partner could not believe the difference in his wife's mood (and I could see a change in his!). On entering the water she was 2 cm dilated and we delivered some 2 hours later.

If you review the maternal theories in Chapter 4, you will see that all the theories played a part in this mother's analgesia with water:

Psychological: a relaxed midwife helped relax both the woman and her partner by breaking the cycle of stress; the environment was also relaxing, with low lights and calming music.

Spiritual: she regressed into herself and changed her mood from stressed to relaxed.

Hormonal: stress hormones were reduced and endorphins and oxytocin increased.

Physiological: water was added to her requirements in both depth and temperature.

The moral of this story – and hundreds more I hear from colleagues all the time – is: don't judge a woman's labour just by how many centimetres dilated she is. By refusing water as an early analgesic you could be seen to be unethical (remember the anaesthetist). It may not be the first – or even, in your clinical judgement, the best – option of analgesia, but it may work for that mother.

When I teach, I ask midwives three questions:

- Do you always judge a mother's labour by invasive vaginal examination?
- Can you tell if a mother is in labour by sitting, watching and palpating contractions?
- If we all did a vaginal examination on the same mother, would we all make her the same dilation?

In most waterbirth situations midwives do not use a set starting point for when to get into the water. We assess mothers individually, deciding with the mother that she is requesting analgesia (her choice being water). Once we believe she is in labour (with or without a vaginal assessment), we will continue to assess labour and if for this particular mother the water has relaxed her too much (contractions reduced), we may suggest she leaves the water and walk around. She can, of course, return to the pool when her contractions re-establish. It is worth reviewing the theories in Chapter 4 regarding enhancing the water environment.

If you wish to read more about patience – watching and listening – there are several good books on the subject: Gaskin (2002, 2008), Davis (2004) and Walsh (2007). This skill has become known as 'masterly inactivity' and papers have been written about the subject; it acts as a foundation for the Royal College of Midwives' *Campaign for Normal Birth* (2006).

Long labour, when mothers are assessed as only niggling, can be very distressing. The description of niggling can make mothers feel that we are not taking their labour pains seriously; I would suggest that a better term is 'spurious labour which nevertheless causes pain and distress and, if it persists for some time, tiredness as well' (RCM 2006). In this situation, it is tempting to augment or induce the labour, which can in itself lead to the cascade of intervention. To assist in breaking this latent labour (Huntingford 1985), water may be used in conjunction with aromatherapy oils to relax the mother. (But be aware that aromatherapy practitioners do not agree whether oils should be used directly in the pool or not; see Burns and Kitzinger 2000 and Tiran and Mack 2000).

Water, of course, is a non-invasive and 'removable' form of analgesia. However, to ensure parents understand that we are taking the mother's labour pains seriously, the terminology we use is vital. Consider which of the following sounds more positive: 'We are going to suggest that you have a bath with some oils', or 'Could we suggest that you use hydrotherapy with relaxing aromatherapy oils in the water?' I was asked to review some notes where a mother complained that she had not been offered any analgesia in labour. On closer inspection, it was found that the mother had been in a bath on the antenatal ward (it was thought that she was in latent labour) and some 2½ hours later was saying that she wanted to push. The head was indeed visible and the midwife supported the mother as she stayed in the water and delivered. Despite having a fast and non-interventionist labour, no drugs, and appropriate monitoring of the fetal heart for latent labour, the one area that was poor was the record keeping. It was documented only that mother was having a bath. Maybe by adding 'for analgesia' or 'as pain relief' this mother's perception could have been altered.

The use of water can be enhanced by the tips offered at the end of the RCM (2006) paper: to block out things that reinforce a sense of time, so no clock or watch in the room; and music rather than radio.

Monitor the condition of mother and baby carefully. Can you identify any factors that may be prolonging labour, such as stress, fear, worry about being believed, fatigue, stressed birth companion? See the theories in Chapter 4.

Vaginal examination under water

It is possible to undertake vaginal examinations under water, with these two provisos. Firstly, ask yourself the fundamental question 'Why am I doing a vaginal examination?' Is it the only way I can assess progress of labour or is it required by my employer (if the latter, you may wish to challenge – but at the right time and right place)? The other concern is protection of the midwife's back – you need to be very careful and this is something I include during my skills drill.

Second Stage

Non-directive pushing

The list of items in Figure 6.2 may assist in giving some ideas as to how to assist with non-directive pushing. As midwives we may well be used to maternal cues to suggest that second stage is approaching. A change in demeanour and mobility is not uncommon; the mother may insist that she wishes to 'go home' or may demand an epidural and even a Caesarean section. However, in my experience, in water maternal cues are more subtle and the ever-vigilant non-intrusive midwife will need to be ready to assist the mother with her birth by picking up these subtle changes.

The second stage of labour is often of great concern to midwives, particularly if you trained during a time of 'controlling the head and guarding the perineum'. Removing my hands was one of the most difficult things to do when I first started waterbirth. The non-touch technique is inherently linked to three main issues: perineal trauma, control over delivery and the newborn's first breath.

In 2006 an article was published by Caroci da costa and Riesco following a study of 70 nulliparous women with 'hands on' (intervention) or 'hands off' (expectant) care. The outcome was that the hands-on technique did not alter or improve the perineal trauma rate. Interestingly, neonatal outcomes were also similar. Although a small study, it does raise the question of whether hands-on management is really to do with perineal trauma or whether it is a question of the health professional having control over the mother at delivery. I never say 'never' to anything in midwifery, and am constantly aware of different circumstances which warrant change in practice, but I do believe that the counter-pressure of the water/mother 'cuddling' or 'cradling' her baby's head does change perineal trauma and impact on a newborn's first breath. See Chapter 7, 'Breathing' and Chapter 9, 'Research'.

- Maternal cues
- Hands off
- Normal mechanism of labour
- Fist breathe

Figure 6.2   Facilitating second stage

Research Relevant to Practice

McCandlish et al. (1998) was a study to see if the HOOP trial can support practice. 5411 women in two units in the period 1994–6 measured perineal pain in the first 24 hours postnatally; they were surveyed at 10 days.

Pain %	'Hands on' care	'Hands off' care
24 hours	3.4%	3.7%
7 days	71.3%	70%
3 months	7%	6.8%

Comment: As you can see from the figures, there are minor differences only.

With waterbirth there is both a physical and a metaphorical hands-off approach, which supports perineal integrity; and of course the research supports reduction in perineal trauma. The hands-on approach is one of the most difficult 'skills' for midwives to move away from.

The normal mechanism of labour may need to be reviewed by practitioners to enhance the care we offer to mothers. When a baby is delivered, the head will crown (chin clears the perineum); it then waits, resituates with internal rotation of shoulders, and delivers. It is important that the midwife understands the 'normal' time frame of delivery and knows when to act if this is delayed. This is particularly important in the case of delay associated with shoulder dystocia – see the 'What if … ?' section later in this chapter. The normal mechanism of labour is beautifully shown in the DVD *A Guide to Waterbirth*, by Ethel Burns, as well as in numerous midwifery texts.

Recently I read an interesting article from an active birth teacher (Lester 2008). She wrote about 'fist breaths' to enhance the effectiveness of bearing down during a contraction in second stage. In the article she continues by saying that it is a tried and tested confidence booster that allows a slow controlled way to push: 'As she feels the contraction beginning, the woman makes a fist with her hand, inhales through her nose, opens her mouth wide, places her fist in her mouth and exhales out over her fist. At the end of the breath out she pauses, relaxes and allows a new breath to come in through her nose.' If you try this yourself you will be amazed at how it seems to release the pelvic floor and encourage the baby to be born.

Perineal integrity

As practitioners we often have to be taught that we need to control the head and guard the perineum during delivery. This traditional method has already been discussed with regard to the HOOP trial. When waterbirths first became popular it seemed that most practitioners felt that the water appeared to stretch the perineum, providing counter-pressure during the delivery. Traditional control therefore appeared redundant. Now we have research (Thni and Mussner 2003; Geisbuehler et al. 2004; Garland 2006a) that confirms that, by facilitating head delivery through vocal support and encouragement, the mother supporting her own perineum and a passive second stage, this style of care is not required in water. The other side of the argument is that controlling the head may cause potential stimuli to the newborn. However, if a mother wishes to guide, cuddle or cradle her baby's head, she is unlikely to do so with such strong touch that the pressure sensors of a newborn will be stimulated.

Perineal integrity also appears to support the fact that fewer tears occur statistically. Those that do occur appear to require delayed suturing. I usually suggest waiting for an hour after leaving the water (unless of course the bleeding is excessive and compromising the mother). I believe that as the tissue is revitalized, haemostasis occurs and because the tear is clean (thanks to the water) I insert fewer sutures. Figure 6.3 is a reminder of these points.

Room environment

This includes the issue of room temperature. Firstly, the room needs to be cool (21–22 °C) to allow the mother's heat to evaporate whilst she is in the pool and for the comfort of the midwife and birth companion. Secondly, in reviewing newborn physiology, it appears to be one factor in the newborn's first breath. If the room is too hot the mother

- Perineal tissues will stretch in water
- Head delivery is facilitated
- Perineal trauma evidence
- Delayed suturing

Figure 6.3   Perineal integrity

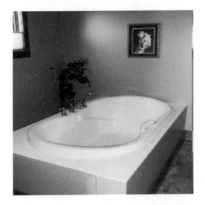 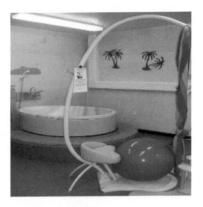

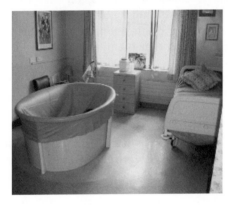

Figure 6.4   Pool room environments

will start to become hyperthermic, with inherent consequences for the fetus. At birth, if the room is not cool, there will be no environmental stimuli to the baby's first breath and it will just lie in its mother's arms, gazing.

Lighting is important within a pool environment. At home it is very easy to change the mood of the room with candles (maybe aromatherapy burners) and other soft lighting rather than just daylight. However, in hospitals and birth centres this may be more challenging. Worldwide there is an amazing diversity of lighting: light mats for the ceiling, Christmas tree lights looped around ceilings/walls/table lamps, electric candles to overhead strip lights. They can all be toned down, which will help to enhance the environment. Figure 6.4 shows a variety of pool room environments.

Third Stage Management: Active versus Physiological

Traditionally, third stage falls into two options: active management with an oxytocic drug or physiological without a drug. However, over the past few years these options have been called into question regarding the issue of mixing managements.

In 2008 Haggertay wrote about giving delayed syntometrine whilst allowing the cord to stop pulsating, thus allowing a further third of blood to be transfused to a newborn. Whilst most people believe this delayed clamping is beneficial to the baby, there appears to be little evidence about the effects of giving delayed syntometrine or indeed any oxytocic drug. Anecdotal evidence from 18 years of waterbirth audits in a hospital in Kent showed that more retained placentas and postpartum haemorrhage occurred when an oxytocic drug was delayed, following a waterbirth and allowing the cord to stop pulsating. Whilst Haggertay concludes that there is no conclusive evidence to recommend delayed oxytocic in conjunction with active third stage, this did not take into account the difference at waterbirth when the cord may well pulsate for longer due to the warm, moist environment. Delay in this situation could be 45–60 minutes. Is this the time to give the delayed oxytocic or should we now proceed with physiological care?

The issue of active or physiological management has been well reviewed. Harris (2001) writes about the introduction of syntometrine in the 1960s and how midwifery textbooks and teaching have focused on the third stage as being 'potentially dangerous for mothers'. Indeed she cites McDonald (1999) in writing, 'for the mother, this [the third stage] has the potential to be the most dangerous stage of labour when the skill and expertise of the midwife will be crucial in facilitating a safe, healthy outcome'.

It is therefore not surprising that widespread use of routine syntometrine has become the norm in Western midwifery. I am well aware that in high-risk mothers the use of an oxytocic may well have profound benefits; however, after a normal low-risk physiological labour and birth (and of course with the mother's consent), I challenge the assumption that all mothers require it routinely.

Another issue to consider with the use of oxytocics is that this necessitates the early clamping and cutting of the cord. This could have an impact on the health and wellbeing of the infant (WHO 1999). Delayed clamping allows the baby to obtain more blood flow from the placenta (approximately 80 ml) (Yao and Lind 1974; Dunn 1985) and this has a positive effect on iron stores. Conversely, many professionals are concerned that delayed clamping and cutting of the cord will cause an increase in physiological jaundice (Woodward et al. 2004).

There are, of course, other issues in developing countries where maternal postpartum haemorrhage (PPH) is still a major cause of maternal mortality. If waterbirth should occur within these settings it would seem prudent to assess the possible benefits of extra blood from the placenta to the newborn versus active management of the third stage. In the last CEMACH report (2003–5), maternal mortality from PPH in the UK was 14 (11 were LSCS deliveries). In developing countries prudent use of an oxytocic drug even after a normal vaginal birth can prove life saving and should not be underestimated in its value.

Effects on the baby of early cord clamping are that it restricts neonatal blood volume and red cell mass at birth (Dawes 1968 cited by Farrar 2009). Whilst it would appear that early clamping reduces physiological jaundice and reduction in iron stores in the first few months of life, any long-term effect is not clear.

It is beyond the scope of this book to discuss all the history, pros and cons, evidence and personal experiences regarding physiological third stage, so I refer the reader to the internet to retrieve articles for discussion and review.

One useful article is Wattis (2001), whose article expands on the history of active management physiology and highlights again the issue that in developing countries active management is officially recommended by WHO to reduce postpartum haemorrhage, which is the commonest cause of maternal death.

Third Stage Options Following a Waterbirth

Option 1: active management

- Risk assessment – interventions performed (ARM, oxytocic, labour, birth position)
- Maternal choice and informed consent
- Early cord clamping and cutting
- Leave water for intramuscular drug
- Non-delayed oxytocic drug:
    o Syntometrine
    o Syntocinon
- Minimal delay when leaving pool
- Hypothetical risk of water emboli if controlled traction attempted under water

- Personal and anecdotal evidence suggests no more than 10 minutes to administration
- Baby to birth companion whilst mother exits pool
- Controlled cord traction as per usual.

Option 2: physiological care

- Risk assessment
- Maternal choice and informed consent
- Cord stop pulsating – may take longer in water (warm and moist environment)
  - o Maternal effort to deliver third stage – see Figure 6.5
  - o As above – mother leaves water – caution with attached newborn!
  - o Cord stop pulsating – clamped and cut – maternal end left clamped – retroplacental clot allows placenta to shear away – in or out of water
  - o Cord stop pulsating – clamped and cut – maternal end left to bleed – not recommended in water as difficult to estimate blood loss (this blood loss is from the fetoplacental circulation and not maternal and thus does not require measuring)
  - o Lotus birth – cord left to stop pulsating – deliver placenta attached and leave to separate physiologically.
- Delay in placental delivery usually classed as greater than one hour – refer to own policy or experience (if mother not bleeding/non-

- Watchful waiting
- Oxytocin release:
  - o warmth
  - o comfort
  - o privacy
  - o no interruptions/ disturbances
  - o feeling unobserved
  - o no bright lights
  - o skin-to-skin contact
  - o breast feeding
  - o nipple stimulation
  - o kisses from partner
- Hydration
- Maternal position

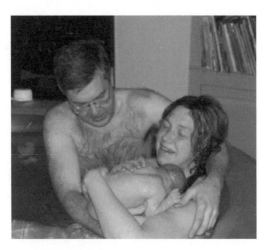

Figure 6.5   Requirements to support physiological third stage

compromised) placenta may take longer than one hour. Consider medical referral and delivery with oxytocic drug per umbilical cord. Traditional or alternative methods of placental delivery are:

- o Dublin or traditional method – pushing down on uterus
- o Crede method – vigorous squeezing

- Both these methods have been abandoned in the UK; however, they may still be practised in some other countries.

Farrar (2009) reminds us that whilst recent papers have recommended the use of syntometrine as the drug of choice for third stage management (Haggertay 2008; Higson 2008), NICE (2007) states that using intramuscular oxytocin has a similar effect on reducing postpartum haemorrhage but without the adverse effects.

Estimating blood loss at delivery

Harris (2001) cites Wickham (1999) in identifying that the total amount of blood loss post placenta delivery is similar in active and physiological third stage; the time frames are different, however. It appears that whilst blood loss at delivery with active management may appear less to begin with, once the action of syntometrine has worn off women may often have a heavy loss on standing once on the postnatal ward. This is borne out by personal correspondence and learnt salient lessons from HCAs (healthcare assistants). They confirm that whilst the active managed blood loss may appear little, when mothers stand up for their shower or bath they often lose a fair amount, which mothers without the injection do not appear to do. In other words, the amount of blood loss is similar – it just occurs at different times at birth and post delivery.

A skill we may need to reintroduce is the accuracy with which we estimate blood loss. Many practitioners have ways of teaching this inaccuracy (when blood goes into bed linen/the bowl/floor etc.). I teach 'games' to students in university and at any clinical opportunity to show how inaccurate we are at estimating blood loss.

There is also the question of an individual woman's ability to cope with blood loss, which may have similar criteria as deciding on supporting physiological third stage. In the UK we are often very poor at using the full definition of a postpartum haemorrhage – that is, blood loss of 500 ml or that which compromises the mother. Over 26 years as a practising midwife, I have seen some mothers compromised by 350 ml and others not compromised by 1000 ml. This is not always dependent on obvious factors but also mode of delivery.

It is the individual mother's ability to cope with blood loss that is the important factor. This issue has been discussed by several authors, with an interesting paper produced by Gyte (1992).

'What if ... ?'

As practitioners we are continually performing ongoing risk assessment during labour and birth. Some changes are major (meconium/slow progress), others are more subtle (physiological heart rate change/maternal pyrexia). Whatever occurs, we make a plan of action and rationalize any change in care with the best evidence, experience and intuition.

This section uses this process to challenge some of the 'What if ... ?' scenarios that may occur with waterbirth.

Maternal choice versus political/professional conflict

In the NHS we are often seen as paternalistic towards clients. In maternity services we have strived to move away from this by offering choice and continuity of care. Building this relationship with mothers has reduced, in some quarters, the conflict of choice that occurred historically. There are still stories of mothers being refused waterbirths even when it has been fully discussed and there are government documents supporting this process. A conflict may then develop between maternal choice and professional stance. I have said a lot in this book about the importance of supporting and working with mothers; the choices they make may not always be the ones that we as professionals would choose, nor based on best evidence – but it is the mother's body and baby and thus her choice. There are still stories in the news about mothers who completely back away from healthcare services, opting out of the system to free birth. In a society where we value and support our maternity services, I find it a very sad reflection on our system that we cannot work through some agreement to provide safe and realistic care.

Poor publicity

Unfortunately, it appears that our media like to cover adverse outcomes regarding poor care. Whilst it is important that this is brought into the public domain, it often serves to frighten women and often does little to truly reflect what actually happened. It is important when adverse outcomes are highlighted that we have an opportunity to reply. With new technology we can now gather information about poor outcomes with waterbirths as soon as they are reported in the media (unlike in 1993, when it took several weeks to gain full information about the death of a Swedish waterbaby after it hit the headlines). In 2007 a waterbaby died in Eire, in 2008 an undiagnosed breech baby was delivered in water and died, and a home waterbaby died in Australia in 2009. These are very severe and sad outcomes but rare; however, they are always the stories which catch the public's eye. Local, national and international organizations will often attempt to provide a balanced view, but as individual practitioners we should be ready to answer a mother's questions. Networking is vital.

Outside criteria

If you review Chapter 10, 'Teaching and Ongoing Education', you will see a learning quiz regarding mothers who may be excluded from using water. I would like to explore a few of the specific mothers and the process undertaken to support the mother with her choice.

Grand multip

In the UK it is not common to be caring for a mother known as a 'grand multip'. Although there are varying definitions in the UK, this is often a mother who has delivered five or more babies, pregnancy losses being included. Usually the reason for caution with this type of mother is with regard to postpartum haemorrhage and serious adverse outcomes, often not quantified by practitioners. In 2008 Reed wrote about two mothers who were both expecting their seventh baby; she wanted to review the evidence regarding risk surrounding grand multiparity. She states that Page and McCandlish (2006) had already reviewed this and concludes, 'I could find no sound evidence to support the belief that grand multiparity on its own is a predictor of severe adverse outcome and the four studies of postpartum haemorrhage indicated no association between grand multiparity and postpartum haemorrhage.'

Certainly when I have encountered a multigravida mother I have researched information about her previous labour and birth history. I would review any relevant information and evidence to assist this mother in making an informed choice.

Group B streptococcus infection

Group B streptococcus infection (GBS) can cause problems of management. It is a silent infection and most mothers who have it are unaware that they are a carrier, unless previous infection or swabs have detected the bacterium. As professionals we have a duty of care to ensure that mothers have informed choice regarding the options for management. The criterion for management varies between hospitals. This may be treatment with prolonged rupture of membranes (itself an issue of what is 'prolonged'), or history of infection in a previous baby, or suspected infection during labour. So parents need to assess all information regarding current guidance on GBS (both the RCOG and the GBS support group give guidance).

In many situations the paediatric team will be happy for a mother to use water, as long as intravenous antibiotics are given (and there are no other risk factors). Some controversy may occur regarding which antibiotics are given, as many mothers have now realized that clindamycin is only required 8-hourly, and is thus less likely to require a second dose in the pool. This fact leads to the wider issue of use of a cannula in the pool. Infection control nurses seem to have two very different views on this – either yes or no! This is confusing for the mother and may also restrict her choice of water. I always recommend that infection control nurses are involved early on in these discussions, so that they can advise on what is the rationale for a negative response, e.g., mothers have no skin lesions, bacteria infections, are fit and healthy, and are perfectly able to deal with a covered cannula in the water. Senior staff may need to be involved in organizing a compromise (for example: cannulate – give IV clindamycin – remove cannula; most mothers will deliver before the next dose or require an intervention – the second dose can be given at 8 hours out of the pool). Everything is possible if carefully negotiated and a clear rationale given; it should, of course, be documented. There is really no consensus regarding a cannula in the pool or not.

Hospital says it does not offer water labour/birth

A hospital might say that it cannot offer water labour/birth because there are no midwives trained for it; the pool is broken; they are too short-staffed; the pool is not always available. These are all too often reasons given within the NHS for not being able to support a mother who wishes to use water for labour or birth. Would we accept these sorts of reasons for not offering an epidural? I think not. And yet while we are seemingly unable to support water use (low risk, low tech), we do support epidurals (high risk, high tech). I leave you to draw your own conclusions.

Leaving water for other analgesia

When I started waterbirth back in 1987, the unit where I worked decided that we would audit any mother who used water for more than an hour. These audits were invaluable in understanding why mothers left the water. We found that 50 per cent of mothers left the water before delivery (reiterated by the Healthcare Commission's *Towards Better Birth*, 2008), of which one-third left for further analgesia options. Many mothers chose to move straight from water to epidurals and all that that implied. We utilized this knowledge to review the theories of hydrotherapy (see Chapter 4), and when we re-audited a year later had dramatically reduced by half the number of mothers who left for further analgesia. The theories helped us to understand that there are many facets of labour (psychological, spiritual, hormonal and physiological) that can be enhanced to support mothers to stay in the water.

As with any type of analgesia, the mother may not find it suits her. Analgesia is not always effective with regard to the quantity and quality that the mother wanted or expected. Expectations are often very high with water, and antenatal preparation is important (see Chapter 5). We can do a lot as practitioners to enhance this analgesia (see Chapter 4). However, despite all attempts to enhance the analgesic qualities of water, some mothers will always leave for further pain relief.

Non-progress in labour

First stage

Another reason for leaving the water in first stage is slow progress of labour. This is always difficult as we are guided by cervical dilation action curves. These do not allow any individuality for a mother's labour. For professionals there are practice issues guided by who and where we work, national guidance (NICE 2007) and professional codes of practice. The individuality of mothers should allow for the ebbs and flows of labour, and acknowledge that it does not follow a set dilation (usually indicated as 1 cm per hour). Once we have established that the water is the right temperature and depth, that the mother is relaxed (reduced stress hormones and increased endorphins and oxytocin) and that we are enhancing the 'aah' effect, most labours will be shorter than land labour (see Chapter 9, 'Research'). However, there will always be mothers whose labours do slow – and these may need to leave the water.

Second stage

Second stage is often not detected until the vertex is visible, although other signs of second stage may be obvious. As second stage is often passive, the length of 'active' pushing may be very short. However, the same safe parameters of practice should be maintained (descent, active contractions, non-compromised mother and fetus). If there are any changes to second stage the mother may need dry land and gravity to assist delivery. It would appear that some mothers just need terra firma (I believe this is sometimes psychological, not just physiological).

Changes to fetal heart rate

Changes to the heart rate may not always be a sign of fetal compromise. The same fetal heart rate change in two mothers may require different management. For example, an early deceleration in a primigravida mother at 2 cm in the pool would require a different risk assessment to a multigravida mother at 9 cm – one may be pathological (primip non-established labour) and the other physiological (multip end first stage).

This is a simple example, but I believe that because many midwives have only practised with continuous monitoring (CTG), they have forgotten normality skills of assessing physiological changes (with risk assessment) that occur in low-risk labours. Midwives who work at home births and midwife-led units are very familiar with these scenarios.

What is important in these situations is the midwife's analysis, action plan and documentation. The action may be 'continue at present and observe, monitoring the fetal heart as the clinical situation dictates'.

Spontaneous rupture of membranes (SRM)

If there are no signs of infection, pyrexia, tachycardia, offensive loss or known risk factors (possibly GBS – see above), and fetal heart auscultation is normal, then there should be no clinical indication not to offer water after SRM. In Chapter 9, you will see that the very few neonatal infections confirm that this is a potential rather than an actual risk. If any changes occur during the labour the suitability of water should be reassessed.

Maternal pyrexia

If careful and robust maternal observations are undertaken prior to pool entry and hourly whilst in the water, there is a low rate of maternal pyrexia. If it does occur, it is vital to establish whether it is physiological. If it is, it should resolve with room/water cooling, extra fluids, change of position (possible use of paracetamol) and ensuring the maternal pulse and fetal heart rate is not raised. The temperature can be rechecked 30 minutes later and if these factors have been reviewed/altered, the mother's temperature should resolve. If it does not resolve, it may be pathological (see influence on fetal compromise and effects of fetal hyperthermia in Chapter 7). In this situation the mother should be asked to leave the water and appropriate action taken.

Water contamination

In my clinical experience this is a fairly rare problem. If there is contamination, it is vital to know what is in the water – blood, meconium or faeces. If there is blood, what stage of labour is the mother at? Bleeding in first stage is probably not normal, and should be very different in amount to SRM or heavy show. Blood at placental separation can appear rather worrying, but in reality a little blood goes a long way. Meconium has already been discussed – probably most mothers will leave the pool. Faeces are unusual as most mothers have a passive second stage and do not evacuate their bowel contents whilst pushing. We do not know the exact reason why this does not occur but it is thought to be partly physiological – firstly, mothers would not normally have their bowels open in a bath, and secondly, the passive second stage with much reduced gravity means there is not the intensity to push as on dry land.

If the water is heavily contaminated, seek the reason and ask the mother to leave the water whilst the pool is emptied, cleaned and restarted. I have only heard of this being required in a handful of situations (see CEMACH 2000–2).

Episiotomy

I have heard of very few situations where an episiotomy has been performed under water, and would not advocate it. As a midwife, I believe an episiotomy would be performed to expedite delivery (if fetal heart rate is very compromised) and in this situation the mother should have left the pool. The debate about whether healing is better in water or on dry land will continue for many years to come. The argument that non-touch delivery and 'poor' vision of the perineum increases the amount of third-degree tears can be dispelled (see Chapter 9).

Shoulder dystocia

It is beyond the scope of this book to discuss shoulder dystocia in any detail, so I will simply highlight warning signs, management in and out of water, and the use of a video for teaching. Shoulder dystocia worries are often given as a reason to exclude or deny a waterbirth to a mother. However, not only is this extremely rare but with clear clinical identification of risk, and action plans and skills drill in place for such an eventuality, these fears can be dispelled.

Warning signs/risk factors for shoulder dystocia:

- maternal age > 35 years
- maternal obesity > 90 kg
- maternal birth weight – macrosomia
- maternal diabetes or gestational diabetes
- fetal size 4 kg +
- pelvic abnormality
- previous shoulder dystocia.

In some of these situations it may be that the mother would be advised to use water for labour (and not birth in the pool). I tend to review delivery in water as the labour progresses.

In labour consider:

- maternal position
- nature of the labour
  - o second stage slow, long gaps in contractions
  - o slow descent/head bobbing
  - o delay with chin clearing the perineum, 'turtle necking'
  - o delay with head rotation
- maternal analgesia – often related to maternal position
- instrumental delivery
- midwife intuition.

Many of these factors are excluded with waterbirth, e.g., instrumental delivery, but all factors need to be considered to accurately assess risk.

The most important factors are slow contractions in second stage (particularly if altered from first stage), slow descent and slow rotation of head. Some of the signs may only be detected by vaginal examination;

however, in combination with other factors they may enable the midwife to risk assess the situation with regard to pending shoulder dystocia.

Dealing with shoulder dystocia:

- risk assess as above
- call for assistance
  - change maternal position in water – deep squat/left lateral
  - ask the mother to stand out of the water – get her to lean over the side of the pool, deep squat out of water, or consider resting her leg on the edge of the pool to open the pelvic diameter.

If you consider tactile stimuli/manoeuvres are required, it is important that full knowledge of newborn's first breath is reviewed. It is therefore not generally considered or recommended that any touch is initiated in the water.

Once the mother has changed position as above it is not uncommon that the rotation of the fetal head can follow very dramatically, and thus the midwife must be ready to catch the baby.

Use of a teaching video

I have only ever seen on video a scenario where there is delay in shoulder delivery. The midwife assesses care and changes the mother's position in the water with a rapid response to very active second stage, slow contractions with long gaps between, slow head descent and delivery of chin. All these factors can be viewed on the US-made video *Born in Water*.

I personally have dealt with four delays with shoulder (I do not say 'dystocia' since a simple change of position assisted delivery and no manoeuvres were required). In two situations the mother remained in the water with a deep squat; in one she stood and leant over the pool; and in the other she was intending to get out but as she lifted her leg to the edge of the pool the baby rotated.

Delay in physiological placental delivery

The main thing with third stage is great patience and watchful care. If you have already discussed physiological management with the mother, she will be aware that this can take up to an hour. From my own experience, discussion with colleagues and through local audit, this seems to be borne out; however, as with all practice issues, there is no set time. I have known placentas take 2 hours (non-compromised mother) and eventually the hormones will release the third stage of labour. Most mothers who wish to have a waterbirth will consent to physiological third stage (see 'Third Stage Options Following a Waterbirth' above).

In my experience the delay simply means that we have to wait – whereas with an oxytocic drug that has not been the management – so masterly inactivity is required. When complications have occurred – PPH or retained placenta – after review the same situation usually occurs: either the mother is not willing to wait any longer or the midwife 'fiddles' or gives a delayed oxytocic drug. I was taught that this 'confuses' the uterus: nature starts the process and at 45–50 minutes, just when the placenta is starting to shear away from the uterine way, an oxytocic is administered.

If the mother and midwife commit to one type of management then – unless she is bleeding severely – we should keep to that management.

Postpartum haemorrhage

The definition of postpartum haemorrhage is blood loss of 500 ml, or any amount which compromises the mother; an excessive amount of bleeding from the genital tract after the birth of the baby. Estimating blood loss is difficult even on dry land, as already discussed, so in water we need to be very vigilant, act swiftly and assess blood loss in more creative ways.

The causes of postpartum haemorrhage are usually described as the 'four Ts': tone, tissues, trauma and thrombin.

Risk factors for postpartum haemorrhage:

- previous history of PPH
- multiple pregnancy
- anaemia
- antepartum haemorrhage
- prolonged labour
- pre-eclampsia
- general anaesthesia
- fibroids
- mismanaged third stage
- retained placenta
- tocolytic drugs

- induced/augmented labour
- inversion of the uterus
- infection.

I believe that mismanaged third stage and not being patient enough are often the main causes of PPH following waterbirth. Understanding the normal physiology and time frames for third stage (audited and usually estimated as one hour) also plays a part. As midwives we need to risk assess the nature of labour throughout and even to the point of birth.

An easy technique that I teach has already been described: use the bottom of the pool as a guide and when you lose sight of the picture/words or mother's legs, recognize that she is bleeding and now is the time to exit the water. You can then manage the PPH out of water – cannulate, give oxytocics, complete third stage delivery, and of course monitor the mother. It should be remembered that a little blood looks a lot in the pool, but with good clinical judgement, experience and early intervention, it should be unnecessary to emergency evacuate with a hoist or net. (As the research in Chapter 9 shows, the number of PPHs is no greater than on dry land, albeit requiring different management.)

Suturing

It is often necessary to wait for approximately one hour after leaving the water before you attempt to suture any perineal trauma, although if the bleeding is severe it must be dealt with immediately. Practitioners seem to agree that if you try to suture too soon, the perineal tissues appear to be water-laden and the tissue is devitalized and difficult to suture; the cellular tissue structure cannot be altered but it does appear that external tissue alters. By waiting an hour, I have found that the tissue has ceased bleeding, is revitalized and needs less suture material in the tear. This is purely observational but may afford further opportunities for reflection.

Water emboli

There are conflicting stories about how and where this theory arose. Michel Odent is the first practitioner to have raised this issue but it is one that to the best of my knowledge has never been seen or documented. When it was first raised back in the 1990s, I investigated this possibility with a physiologist and university physics laboratory. Both came to similar conclusions: they could only envisage two occasions when a water embolus could occur: if a mother straddles a jacuzzi outlet; or if you attempt to deliver the placenta with controlled cord traction under water. (Physiological management of third stage is acceptable and safe as it is passive not active.)

Maternal collapse – fainting, PPH or cardiac emergency

In my experience these are very different issues. Fainting tends to occur because the room has become too hot. Collapse due to PPH should have been detected before the point in time when a mother needs emergency evacuation – see above. The only time that emergency evacuation should occur (and to the best of my knowledge has never occurred) is when the mother suffers an out-of-the-blue cardiac arrest. In the UK this would be the only time that midwives would need the support of moving and handling staff. A new DVD is planned to show midwives how to evacuate in this situation. The photograph in Figure 6.6 shows the principles of the manoeuvre, which should be practised as part of your skills drill.

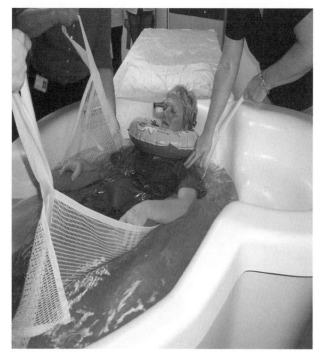

Figure 6.6 Emergency evacuation, using a Silverlea net

Questions for Discussion and Reflection

- Do you feel confident and competent to support a mother with physiological underwater third stage?
- Do you have the opportunity to undertake skills drills for all aspects of waterbirth?

7

Breathing

In Utero Consciousness

This may seem an unusual way to start a chapter regarding the first breath, but I would like to share some thoughts on *in utero* consciousness. When does a fetus take on a life of its own? The anti-abortionist lobby would say that he/she has an entity of its own at conception; others will say from viability; others from birth. In 1979 Wambach attempted to answer some of these questions through a study of 750 people who were put under hypnosis. These people were asked to recall their memories of *in utero* life, labour and delivery, which makes fascinating reading. This small study appears to support the theory that the baby is a separate entity early *in utero* and probably by 6 months. Many of the subjects reported that they found their births a time of great sadness and that on emerging from the womb 'reported a rush of physical sensations ... that was disturbing and unpleasant'.

Many women say that they have an attachment to their baby when they first feel it move or towards the time that their baby is due. Why is this important to waterbirth? Well, a mother's consciousness of her baby can be enhanced by water early on in pregnancy: being aware of the baby's reaction to the antenatal swimming and relaxing, his perception of relaxation; there should be a reduction of stress hormones and a surge of endorphins. We stress to mothers the importance of *in utero* life, advising avoidance of harmful substances (alcohol and drugs), a well-balanced diet and a loving environment. Delivering into a quiet and calm, warm, welcoming pool is essential to the birth environment. We encourage skin-to-skin contact, and promote breast feeding and time together as a new family with minimal disturbance.

Water is an environment that the baby is familiar with; it has supported and cradled him for 9 months. It is an environment that is enabling him to unfold and explore slowly as the first breath and adaptation to extra-uterine life commences.

Verny (1987) believes that there is a fine interplay between mother and baby. He believes that the vulnerability of a baby is highlighted by the bombardment of stimuli which trigger respiration and the first breath. Is that first cry one of joy or a way of communicating distress and subsequently his needs? Verny writes: 'Even in the best circumstances, birth reverberates through the child's body like a seismic shock of earthquake proportions.' Although oxytocin is said to have an amnesiac effect, nothing, according to Verny, will escape the baby's memory – every feeling and every movement is remembered.

Knowing some of this background, it is not surprising that mothers seek a gentle birth for their babies, and that as midwives we engage in providing a quiet, calm birth environment.

Effects of Hormones

In utero babies are subjected to increasing amounts of circulating hormones to promote development and growth. Crossover of adrenal steroids via the placenta is said by Pearce (1977) to leave the fetus and infant 'locked in a free floating anxiety'. Stress hormones are 20 times higher in a baby than in an adult, and 10 times higher in a mother giving birth. The increase in hormone levels and the inherent normal physiological hypoxaemia of labour is transient. Physiologically the fetus has adaptive mechanisms to counteract this, such as high levels of fetal haemoglobin (fHb) with its affinity for oxygen. Stress hormones counteract the effects of oxygen deprivation by increasing blood pressure and heart output, especially to the vital organs. In more recent times other authors have highlighted this physiological process (see Balaskas and Gordon 1992).

Fetal Heat Adaptation

The fetus is very dependent on his mother for heat transfer. Temperature control is based on heat transfer via a pathway between mother and baby (Appendix 3 illustrates this in detail; Power 1989). The placenta acts as a heat exchanger between mother and fetus, and assists in maintaining the fetal temperature at 0.5–1.0 °C above the mother's. This balance of heat control is dependent upon the temperature of the surrounding maternal tissues. Heat accumulates in the fetal body and surrounding amniotic fluids. The differential between the mother's and baby's temperature allows this heat to pass to the mother through the umbilical circulation. The fetal skin, amniotic fluid, and placenta and uterine wall are all reliant on the mother's heat control systems. A rise in maternal and fetal temperatures shows an immediate increase in fetal heart rate.

A similar situation may also occur with an epidural; indeed there has been an increasing body of evidence which conflicts regarding the impact of hyperthermia on cerebral injury or ischaemia (Macaulay et al. 1992; Perlman 2006; Palanisamy et al. 2007). What does seem clear is that a rise in maternal temperature whether with epidural or in water – with an unknown aetiology – is to be avoided wherever possible.

The fetus is in a warm, thermoneutral environment, and its own fetal metabolism produces minimal active thermogenesis or heat production *in utero*.

At birth, the newborn thermal regulation is poor. The baby has reduced subcutaneous layers of fat and heat loss is said to be four times higher than in the adult. This naturally has implications for postnatal care following waterbirth. Heat loss through evaporation is reduced in the presence of vernix and the fine thermal control can be further affected by hypoxia and hypoglycaemia – thus low-risk newborns that have not suffered hypoxia and have early feeding encounter minimal reactions. The effects of cold on the newborn, with temperatures between 27 °C and 32 °C in the presence of hypoglycaemia, can cause a higher incidence of pulmonary haemorrhage. Clinically, this means we should ensure the baby is dried and kept warm, with no draughts in the pool environment, skin to skin being the obvious position for the baby. If mother and baby are in the water, the temperature must be monitored.

Fetal Perspective on Waterbirth

A quote from some 35 years ago still seems as relevant today as it was all those years ago: 'The simple fact is that as soon as a child is born he starts to cry and how bitterly. And although this is strange, it is the one thing that delights everyone there … how beautifully my baby cries, exclaims the happy mother, thrilled and amazed that something so little can make so much noise' (Leboyer 1975). Leboyer's intention was twofold: not to cause the baby unnecessary distress, and to welcome him or her into the world in as comfortable a way as possible with a bath in warm water.

Here is a thought on how our knowledge has altered in the past 100 years. In 1909 Giles wrote (cited in Channel 4's film *Brave New Babies*):

The senses lie dormant when the child is in the womb: in the darkness and quiet in its aquatic existence it sees nothing, hears nothing; it neither tastes nor smells; no variations of temperature occur to stimulate it and even the sense of touch is hardly called into play because the fluid, in which it lies, presses on it evenly and without variation.

Is crying just a way of showing us that all his reflexes and senses are working, or is it the baby trying to express something else – pain, suffering or sorrow?

We have altered birth rooms, making them more home-like, with warm, calm, low lighting, and soft noises only from a welcoming family. We have learnt so much about the *in utero* senses of a baby; we believe they are very aware of their surroundings – indeed scans have given us the opportunity to venture into that environment. It is therefore not surprising that waterbabies, born into warmth, quiet and calm, and delivered and brought to the water surface by hands that are welcoming – often the mother's – are calm and quiet themselves.

Leboyer (1975) also said:

We were wondering about how best to prepare the child ... now we see it's not the child who needs to be prepared. *It is ourselves* [my italics]. It is our eyes that need to be open, our blindness that has to stop. If we used just a little intelligence how simple things could be.

Waterbirths have often been introduced into areas of high medical intervention. Knowledge about maternal and fetal interplay has shown us that the two cannot be separated; there is a strong interdependent reaction between mother and baby.

Fetal Protection against Inhalation of Water

There is a mechanism, shown in Figure 7.1, which is believed to assist in the initial suppression and then first breath of the newborn (see Harper 2005). The figure identifies some of those factors, commencing with the effect of prostaglandin inhibition, and normal fetal breathing movements (FBM) from 10 weeks' gestation. We know the fetus *in utero* practises a regular and rhythmic pattern of movements of intercostal and diaphragm muscles. Twenty-four to forty-eight hours before the onset of spontaneous labour the fetus has an increase in prostaglandin E2 levels from the placenta, which causes a slowing or stopping of these 'practice breaths'. When the baby is born these levels

In utero breathing inhibitors:

1. Prostaglandin E2 effect
   - FBM start at 10/40 and occur 40% of the time *in utero*
   - 24–48 hours prior to labour starting FBM decrease
2. Alveoli lung fluid – maintained by osmotic pressure – fluid remains in upper airways
3. Mild hypoxia during birth – conserves oxygen – decreases FBM
4. Dive reflex – chemoreceptors protect airway

Figure 7.1   First breath, from womb to room

are still high and thus do not stimulate breath movement; therefore the first inhibitory response engages.

It would be interesting to know what impact induction of a labour has on these fetal breathing movements. In my experience, many units exclude women who are being induced (including post-maturity) from using water. If this mechanism is followed through, it may be that they are right but for the wrong reason. If the normal decrease of fetal breathing movements has not occurred – due to induced labour – is there a greater risk of the fetus attempting to 'breathe' underwater? From personal experience teaching around the world, I would say this does not appear to be a problem, and many units do offer water to induced mothers.

The other factors listed all play an important part in the physiology of first breath; these are described more fully below in this chapter.

In 1995, at the first international waterbirth conference, Dr Paul Johnson (physiologist at the John Radcliffe Hospital, Oxford) presented his views on the inhibition of the first breath in water. He stated views and ideas which represented the first main theory about what many practitioners had seen in practice. He stated that breathing is inhibited through natural physiological processes, including hormones (prostaglandins, progesterone, adenosine and endorphins) released from the placenta and a low metabolic rate.

All babies have an inbuilt inhibitory response due to the fact that they are experiencing a mild hypoxia during labour. This causes apnoea (the absence of breathing) and swallowing, not breathing or gasping. This process is further supported by the large number of chemoreceptors (thought to be five times more than found on the whole of the tongue) found in the larynx of the newborn, which are said to facilitate the baby to recognize which fluids can be swallowed – and thus close the glottis – or which should be inhaled. This autonomic reflex is built into newborns to assist them with breast feeding and remains intact for some 6–9 months, after which it seems to disappear (Harper 2000).

Johnson (1996) states that the fetal larynx response is similar to a reduced diving response of bradycardia and hypertension. It is only when severe fetal hypoxia occurs that fetal breathing is inhibited (if terminal, then gasping occurs).

The analogies are seen in clinical practice every day on a basic level. Consider what happens when you give a baby its first formula feed. Does it not gag or spit it out? Could this be the chemoreceptor reaction to a substance which is not known to them and they are unsure whether to swallow or inhale?

Another analogy is with regard to meconium. Why is it that babies who have meconium in labour do not then all present at birth with meconium aspiration? We believe it is because the chemoreceptors have a high affinity to an alien substance (meconium) and therefore unless there is severe hypoxia they will protect the baby's larynx. If no hypoxia is present the chemoreceptors will protect the baby's larynx and thus it does not inhale. This response can be overridden and may explain some of the so-called 'drownings' of recent years, as they were referred to in national newspapers in 1993.

Research Relevant to Practice

Johnson (1996) explores the multifactorial stimulus to newborn respiration and looks at why there is a 'protective' mechanism in waterbirth. He highlights five inhibitions in water: endocrine (endorphin production), ambient temperature of water (37 °C), metabolism – thermogenesis, chemical – hypoxia, and airway chemoreceptors.

- A baby practises breathing movements *in utero* early in pregnancy, which influences lung development. Movement of the diaphragm and chest stimulate lung and alveolar development. *In utero* lungs are already filled with fluid – so no aspiration. Lung fluid is absorbed when the first breath is taken and usually completed by 6 hours after birth.
- Prostaglandin E2 produced by the placenta inhibits brain functions including breathing, which contributes to cessation of breathing movements 48 hours before the start of labour. 24–48 hours before the onset of spontaneous labour the fetus experiences a

notable increase in prostaglandin E2 levels from the placenta. The rise in hormone levels softens the cervix, makes the uterus more susceptible to oxytocin and causes a slowing or stopping of fetal breathing movements.

- Dive reflex. The umbilical cord pulsates – no reflex bradycardia occurs. It is important to assess fetal heart rate and time scales for head/body delivery.
- Apnoea (cessation of breathing) occurs in the expiratory position with closure of larynx triggered by receptors in the skin transmitted via the trigeminus nerve. If the reflex continues to work, reflex bradycardia commences – change in heart minute volume in favour of blood distribution to essential organs.
- The dive reflex (see Figure 7.2) occurs due to high concentration of chemoreceptors at the back of the baby's larynx which allows it to close to any abnormal substance, closes the glottis and stops fluid passing into the respiratory tract. This mechanism is similar to how a baby breast feeds (and prevents food from regurgitating) and is present until the baby is about 6–9 months old, when the reflex disappears. There is some debate that this reflex may get weaker the more stimulation it receives (therefore babies are not re-submerged). A compromised newborn has the potential for gasping before the nose and mouth have been delivered.
- Mild hypoxaemia occurs during labour – less oxygen being received by newborns as labour starts. This is a normal state that babies cope with *in utero*. The adaptive process allows babies to cope and causes apnoea (absence of breathing) and swallowing, not breathing or gasping.

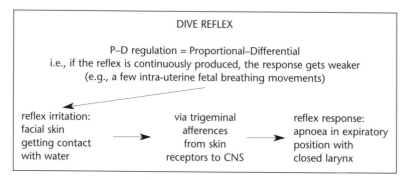

Figure 7.2 Diagram of the dive reflex (adapted from Burke 1985)

Initiation of the First Breath

Box 7.1 summarizes the factors which stimulate the first breath in the newborn on dry land. It shows a number of stimuli rather than just one to 'trigger' the first breath.

Box 7.1 Factors that stimulate the first breath

TRIGGER IN AIR	WATERBIRTH MIMIC
Environment	
Room temperature 21–22 °C	Water temperature 37–37.5 °C
Gravity	
Full force of gravity	Reduced gravity in water
Pressure sensors	
Delivery technique	Non-touch technique
Gravity	Reduced gravity
Touch	
Delivery technique	Non-touch technique
Suctioning	No suctioning
Sound	
Sounds of delivery	Muffled in water
Chemoreceptors	
Stimulated by labour hypoxaemia	Healthy baby
Clamping and cutting cord	No clamping or cutting
	Recognition of fluids
Closure of temporary structures	
Changes to CSF pressure	Stimulation sequence in air
Clamping and cutting of cord	
Alveoli fluid absorbed	
Head's reflex	
Triggered by lung expansion	Occurs with first breath

Adapted from Burke (1985)

Environment

In many countries around the world it is still thought correct management to deliver the baby into normal adult body temperature (37 °C). Cooling of air temperature by as little as 1–2 °C will trigger fetal breathing and coordinate the diaphragmatic muscles (Mackay 2001).

These temperature changes are minimal as birth occurs in normal adult body temperature. However, there are many reports of ocean births and controlled cool waterbirths where water temperature is not measured and babies are born into relatively cool water, apparently without any adverse outcomes. The most notable proponent of the cool waterbirth is Cornelia Enning, a German midwife (see her adapted Apgar score below). Enning, as others, does not believe that the water temperature plays as large a part in stimulation as I do. Even though we practise very differently, both have large numbers of audited births.

At present in the UK and most other waterbirth centres, normal adult body temperature is that which is offered for waterbirth. In 2002 Harper raised the question of water temperature at the time of birth and wondered whether, like Russia, Germany and Eastern European countries where lower temperatures are used, we should revisit our guidelines.

Reports suggest that babies born into cooler temperatures have a faster adaptation to their new dry land environment. I do not believe that the birth water temperature issue is yet resolved, but for UK practitioners the RCOG/RCM guidelines (2006) still recommend normal adult body temperature for birth.

Gravity

When a baby is born in water the full force of gravity is reduced (assuming the baby is completely underwater – hence water depth is important). Gravity stimulates the baby through pressure sensors, particularly on the top of its head, but there are many pressure sensors throughout our bodies. These will not be triggered until the baby leaves the water.

Pressure sensors

Zimmerman (1993) writes that the hydrostatic pressure present during a waterbirth is less than on dry land, therefore there is no need for *traditional* control of the fetal head.

This is something which midwives may find difficult to give up doing. As far back as 1914 (Fairbairn), midwifery textbooks were advocating controlling the head and guarding the perineum. However, in waterbirths we aim to provide a non-touch technique. Many mothers do choose to feel their baby's head during delivery, but I say to midwives and mothers that this is more like 'cradling' or 'cuddling' their baby's head rather than 'controlling', the way that tradition has taught midwives.

Touch

One issue which often arises with waterbirth is that of non-touch technique. In this chapter we are reviewing that in light of newborn physiology; however, it should also be reviewed with reference to perineal trauma (see Chapter 6).

Sound

We now appear to agree that babies have a perception of sound *in utero*. Loud noises stimulate them, calm music or mother's voice can soothe them. Under water any sounds that are present are muffled until the ear leaves the water. Another interesting fact is that in pool rooms, possibly due to the calm environment, there is very little noise from midwife or birth companion. The first noise the baby should hear is that of its mother welcoming him to the world.

Chemoreceptors

This is a strong chemosensitive region which provokes a strong dive reflex (see the section on the dive reflex, above).

Babies enter the world in a degree of hypoxia – low oxygen – which occurs during labour; however, most babies are capable of dealing with this hypoxia and compensate. Hypoxia causes apnoea and swallowing, not breathing or gasping. If the hypoxia is severe and prolonged, the baby may show changes to the heart rate, which the midwife needs to establish is pathological and not physiological. If the baby was delivered underwater during this pathological event it may gasp when born and subsequently inhale water.

Closure of temporary structures

Once the newborn has contact with the air the shunts in the baby's heart, which bypass the lungs, close; fetal circulation changes, and the lungs experience oxygen for the first time.

I remember being taught as a student midwife that the first breath was dependent on the pressure in the vagina squeezing all the lung fluid out during delivery. We now know there is no vacuum created during delivery, and this action has little bearing on newborn breathing.

The lung fluid is automatically pushed out into the vascular system from the pressure of the pulmonary circulation, thus increasing the blood volume by some 20 per cent. The lymphatic system absorbs the rest of the fluid through the interstitial spaces in the alveolar epithelium due to adrenaline. This process can take anywhere from 6 to 48 hours and is vital for the baby's health (Mackay 2001; Harper 2005).

Water is a hypotonic solution whilst lung fluid is hypertonic. Hypertonic fluids are denser than hypotonic fluids, so even if water did enter the lungs these fluids could not merge with a denser fluid.

Head's reflex

This is a paradoxical effect whereby the newborn has a vagal stimulus which is triggered by inspiration (Widdicombe 2004). Cross further investigated Head's reflex in 1961, describing the vigorous inspiratory movements which we see at birth. The cry of birth that is often heard on dry land very early in the baby's first breath often does not occur following waterbirth; this is due to an altered physiology for a few moments in time. The cry of birth is actually an expiratory activity. Midwives often need to relearn the first breath physiology. We often miss Head's reflex on dry land since the baby receives some stimuli before full delivery (touch, light, sound), sometimes attempting to cry on the perineum. It is very important to find out if a previous baby did this at birth, as multigravid mothers may be anxious if they remember this.

This physiology may go some way to explain why waterbabies appear blue when first born. Johnson (1996) writes:

> Of course a baby delivered in this fashion does not receive the multiple stimuli to breathe simultaneously as would occur in most conventional births – cool air, light, sound, gravity. It is therefore likely that the onset of air breathing will commence quietly without crying and thus effective gas exchange may be slower to be established. It might be anticipated that infants may be more often blue or cyanotic for longer periods.

We are aware that several stimuli initiate the first breath of the baby when leaving water (Hamed et al. 1967; Burke 1985). However, the physiology even prior to birth plays a part in this sequence of events, as has been described (see Figure 7.3).

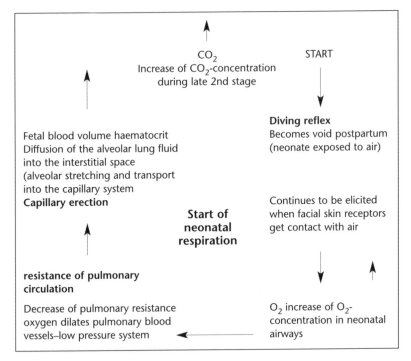

Figure 7.3 Diagram of neonatal respiration

Apgar Scoring after Waterbirth

In 1953 when Virginia Apgar introduced her scoring system it was heralded as a systematic method for assessing newborn condition at birth. Over the years it has been challenged but is still widely used and understood by practitioners around the world. One such paper published in 2004 by Lopriore et al. wrote about problems with inter-observer variation. Although this article mainly deals with newborns who require resuscitation, the relevance is just as important when assessing waterbabies. It is not uncommon for waterbabies to have Apgar scores of 10 at one minute. Clinically, it is vital that one full minute is allowed to elapse before we assess Apgar scores. When this is allowed to occur inter-observer variations can be reduced, true one-minute Apgar scores are recorded, and as midwives we can transfer this knowledge to dry land births.

There are many variables that can influence Apgar scores – gestational age, maternal analgesia and subjective scoring by the practitioner.

The whole Apgar score is debatable in its value in long-term prediction of morbidity (Crozier and Sinclair 1999). There appears to be discrepancy in the correlation between clinical picture, fetal heart rate changes, Apgar scores, cord pH and long-term sequelae.

How often as midwives have we attended an emergency LSCS, undertaken on one or more clinical factors (changes to heart rate and meconium), only to deliver a baby with good Apgar scores/cord pH? Even when we review all factors and use our best clinical skills, the data do not always prove an exact science. Conversely, occasionally babies who should be delivered in good condition require resuscitation when there were no obvious risk factors. Maybe new technology for high-risk mothers/babies using ECG could prove more beneficial, or maybe we need a back-to-basics assessment.

However, for waterbabies the biggest challenge is to ensure that the Apgar score is recorded at one minute to allow the first breath physiology to occur. Remember that the physiology is delayed and occurs at a slower pace than on dry land, when all stimuli occur simultaneously. A minute is a long time for the baby to initiate his first breath, but give him time – he will gaze at you, have good muscle tone, open eyes and a normal heart rate, but he will remain blue for a few extra seconds and until the Head's reflex commences at 45–50 seconds.

The clinical implications for Apgar score – the importance of one minute not 45 seconds

The shortfalls of Apgar scoring were highlighted in a survey (Lopriore et al. 2004) undertaken in Holland in 2004. Several cases of Apgar scoring (babies needing resuscitation/intubation) were identified to 166 paediatric professionals, who were asked to assess and record the score. Scores varied widely, which supports what is found in clinical practice – that as professionals we may not always agree with each other's assessment. With waterbabies it is vital that we do wait a full minute (make use of a second midwife/student to ensure one minute is actually measured). If you do not ensure Apgars at one minute it is possible that you will record Apgars of 7/8 – and then, quite rightly, paediatricians will ask why you are getting 'low' scores with low-risk babies.

Enning (2007) goes one step further by identifying a new Apgar score, which she believes can be used with waterbirths and is more accurate with the delayed first breath physiology (see Table 7.1).

Table 7.1 Apgar score (adapted from Enning 2007)

Finding	0	1	2	Record at 1, 5, 10 mins
Pulse	Absent	< 100	> 100	
Respiratory effort	Absent	Irregular	Regular	
Lung fluid expulsion reflex (LFER)	Absent	Chest movement	Open mouth	
Appearance (colour)	Pale/blue	Extremities blue	Pink all over	
Activity (muscle tone)	Floppy	Grasp reflex (hands and feet)	Swimming movements	
Grimace (eye movement)	Closed	Briefly open	Focusing blinking	

Questions to ask about Apgar scores

Here are some questions we can usefully ask ourselves (drawn from Simkin 1986; Johnson 1996; Harper 2005):

- Why do babies not breathe underwater and, indeed, what causes them to take their first breath in air?
- What are the practical and physiological implications of complications in water? What can we safely do when they occur?
- What care do we offer newborns after delivery?
- What knowledge do parents have about physiology and first breath?

In 2005 Kassim et al. wrote about some cases of respiratory distress following adverse effects of aspiration of water – they stress that unrecognized hypoxia may cause a newborn to gasp under water. Diligent risk assessment, monitoring of the fetal heart, colour of liquor and midwife's intuition all play a part in foreseeing complications. In my experience, poor outcomes may be associated with waterbirth, so when you review any adverse outcomes, reflect on clinical assessment and robust clinical care as a possible association. I have been taught by a paediatrician that 'water may be an association but is highly unlikely to be a causation'.

Research Relevant to Practice

Eckert et al. (2001) carried out a randomized control trial of 274 women in Adelaide, NSW, who were in water in the first stage of labour, compared with dry land births.

Results:

Pharmacological analgesia – same

IOL/augmentation, perineal trauma, length of labour, mode of delivery – same results

Neonatal outcomes: birth weight, Apgar scores, meconium-stained liquor, cord pH – not statistically different

Bath babies did require more resuscitation: 19% versus 13%, classed as 7 at one minute – Apgars balance out in both groups at 5 minutes

Client satisfaction – same

Comment: Clinical assessment by midwives undertaking waterbirths – important to assess Apgar at one minute and not earlier.

Care of the newborn

Once the baby has gently emerged from the water and the Apgar score has been accurately assessed (and of course any resuscitation initiated), the baby is bought to the mother's arms. Bringing the baby to the surface slowly allows time to ensure cord entanglement and integrity is normal. You can gently unravel any cord around the head, body or limbs, and ensure the cord is long enough to place into his/her mother's arms. It is really good if the mother or birth companion lifts the baby out but not all parents wish to do this, and the 'expectant' midwife should be ready to assist.

Depending on the mother's position in the pool, there may need to be a change in position for receiving the baby – if she is semi-recumbent place the baby on her knee area or chest; if she is squatting, the baby comes into her arms or head just above water; if she is kneeling, place the baby at her chest. It is important to remember that only the baby's head needs to emerge from the water to initiate the first breath. The mother can then change position to facilitate skin-to-skin contact.

It is important to keep the baby warm, skin to skin being the most obvious form of thermoregulation (see Figure 7.4). Also ensure that there are no draughts and, if towels are placed around mother and baby, make sure they do not drape in the water and get damp.

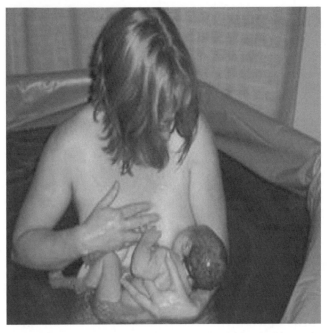

Figure 7.4   Skin-to-skin contact – first contact and feed with mother, Kate

In my experience, generally babies do not require any extra observations, although this will need to reflect your own normal immediate care of the newborn.

Cord clamping is dealt with in Chapter 6.

Benefits of Waterbirth to the Baby

Despite the baby being such an important part in waterbirth, very little is written about benefits to him; and what is written is not substantiated and tends to be based on anecdotal evidence and birth stories (see Chapter 9). Below are some of the perceived benefits recorded by practitioners and parents.

- enhanced fetal oxygenation (improved blood flow to baby due to better blood circulation in mother)
- gentler transition (Ponette 1996)
- less birth trauma (Ponette 1996)

- thermoneutral water temperature for baby (Mackay 2001)
- reduction of sensory stimuli (Leboyer 1975)
- reduction in gravity 'shock' of birth (Tjarkovsky cited in Sidenbladh 1983)
- relaxed and peaceful environment – (Lichy and Herzberg 1993)
- skin-to-skin contact – (Garland 2000a)

The benefits of early swimming in newborns (Smirnov 2002) are:

- improved physical growth
- improved cognitive functions – memory, attention, imitative construction.

As the baby emerges it is often 'caught' by either parent or midwife. We do not believe that the midwife needs to bring the baby to the surface – parents should be encouraged to lift their own babies to the surface. The baby can unwrap itself and has freedom to move in the water with the recognition of a warm watery environment, a familiar place to discover the new world. Light is dimmed and sounds are quiet, and the first welcoming signs a baby receives are those from his/her parents. This truly gentle form of birth is explored by Harper (2005).

Research Relevant to Practice

A study by Geissbuehler et al. (2002) in Switzerland studied neonatal and maternal outcomes in 10,775 births.

Neonatal outcomes	Average results	
	Water – 3162	Land – 5272
Arterial pH	7.3	7.27
Venous pH	7.4	7.37
Apgar one minute	8	8
Apgar at 5 minutes	9	9
Apgar at 10 minutes	9	9
RDS	7	56
NICU	9	42
Infection	17	55
Febrile > 38 °C	8	28

A smaller study compared maternal and neonatal temperatures. There were 30 waterbirths and 17 land births.

Maternal temperature	Water °C	Land °C
O/A	36.3	36.4
Bath begin	36.7 maternal	
Birth	36.9	36.3
End of bath	36.9	
1 hour after birth	36.9	36.6
Discharge	36.7	36

Neonate temperature	Water °C	Land °C
15 minutes after birth	36.9	36.8
60 minutes	36.9	37
At discharge	36.9	36.8

There have been reports from Sweden, Taiwan, New Zealand, France, United Kingdom and Ireland of poor outcomes following waterbirth. When these situations appear in the press (usually via a Google alert – a very useful way of keeping abreast of waterbirth issues), I do several things. Firstly, if possible (and with an appropriate time gap) I would aim to contact the unit to see if I can offer any professional support or advice. I try to find out as much information as possible – was it unexplained, or a skills/professional issue? I repeat the phrase here that was used by a consultant paediatrician some years ago: 'the water may be an association but is highly unlikely to be a causation'.

The chief paediatrician at Ostend, Dr M. Naert, wrote in Ponette (1999):

> all the prejudices appeared to be unfounded. You can see that the child, who is born underwater, feels good in it. Until now, I have never found any complication with the new born as a result of the underwater birth, no infection, no aspiration of the bathwater ... I do see an intense experiencing of the birth, by both the parents and the child. There is a certain decline in the number of medical interventions. The mother and her baby can only benefit from this.

Gilbert and Tookey (1999) and Nikoderm (2004) both identified some possible complications following waterbirths. Although the Cochrane review (Nikoderm) revealed a tendency towards lower Apgars, lower pH at birth and increased rates of neonatal infection, this was not the finding of the earlier paper by Gilbert. The results of many audits and well-recognized papers are reported upon in Chapter 9 of this book. Both authors take care to point out that these figures may mask specific complications of waterbirth, including water aspiration and snapped umbilical cord. Whilst I agree that back in 1999 under-reporting may have occurred, with the plethora of government support in the UK, such as clinical governance and risk management processes, I believe that all complications of all births are now well documented and more importantly investigated and acted upon.

In 2005 Kassim et al. wrote about an incident whereby a low-risk baby was diagnosed with respiratory distress following a waterbirth. The baby started to 'grunt' at one hour of age and was transferred to the neonatal unit at 3 hours. X-ray examination showed changes consistent with aspiration of pool water. The infection screen was negative and the baby was discharged; a follow-up check at 3 months showed no symptoms. We must ask ourselves why this situation might have occurred.

'What if ... ?' The Fetal Perspective

With any complication midwives need to ensure they have the skills for dealing with the problem. However, this starts early in care – recognition of previous problems (shoulder dystocia), current changes during labour (such as slow second stage) and events which may happen at delivery (nuchal cord). Water is not the panacea for all evils, and whatever can happen on dry land can happen in water. Our skills are detection, recognition and management. I believe there are some different issues with regard to fetal/newborn problems than those already dealt with in the section in Chapter 6 on 'What if ... ?' For example:

- Are there physiological areas that need to be highlighted: for example, what is the impact of clamping and cutting the cord under water?
- Are the mechanisms of labour altered by the complication?
- Would you have time to empty the pool in an emergency, bearing in mind that most pools take 15–60 minutes to empty? Is it quicker to ask the mother to stand out of the water?
- Will risk managers and colleagues be supportive if unforeseen complications arise?

Changes to fetal heart rate

The NICE intrapartum guidelines (2007) recommend intermittent auscultation for low-risk mothers.

Intermittent auscultation with underwater soniciads is suitable; they give both a visual and a digital display. If there are any changes to the fetal heart rate it is vital that we assess whether these are physiological (due to compression and progress of labour – early decelerations) or pathological (due to fetal compromise – late decelerations). I am aware that this is rather simplistic since we also need to take account of parity, length of labour, stage of labour, progress, maternal position analgesia used, using our clinical skills, intuition and experience. It is not an easy decision but one which utilizes many skills. If the fetal heart changes and is assessed as pathological then the mother should be asked to leave the pool, or, if delivery is imminent, then to stand out of the water, as leaving the pool at this stage may be very difficult.

Meconium-stained liquor

Despite the ongoing debate regarding meconium-stained liquor, it appears that most practitioners will view this as a potential sign of fetal compromise. It is estimated that meconium is present in 15 per cent of all deliveries and in 40 per cent of post-mature labours. Most practitioners would therefore suggest that the mother leaves the water. However, the challenge is to know whether this is physiological or pathological meconium – do we manage both of these scenarios in the same way? How should we manage the primigravida mother – low risk – with meconium on SRM at 3 cm, or the multigravida mother who is low risk but post mature, who at 9 cm shows meconium? Many midwives would manage both mothers the same – leave the water; others would leave the multip to deliver or have a 'wait and review' management. Where meconium is 'graded', management may also depend on what consistency the meconium presents with. It is not an easy decision.

Nuchal cord

During a normal birth a nuchal cord, which is said to be present in approximately 25 per cent of births, may increase the likelihood of fetal bradycardia and variable decelerations. Handling the cord to loop it over the baby's head will involve touching and stretching the cord, stimulating umbilical arteries to vasoconstrict. The premature gasp that this handling may initiate is not thought to be a problem on dry land. However, at a waterbirth this premature gasp may carry the associated risks of water inhalation. This, of course, would be further compounded and complicated by a tight cord, which the midwife may traditionally have clamped and cut. These courses of action have been questioned by waterbirth midwives for many years; indeed in clinical guidelines and in my teaching throughout my years of experience, I have always stressed that to prevent the initiation of respiration one should never clamp and cut the cord under water. It is, I believe, becoming less common for midwives to feel for the cord rather than loop it over the head.

The level of research surrounding the practice of nuchal cord management appears somewhat lacking. Medico-legal reviews have identified that clamping and cutting of the cord 'is dangerous and should be avoided ... [it] poses a risk management problem for practitioners and Trusts' (Reed 2007). As midwives we should be undertaking practice that has a sound evidence base and only use a skill for which there has been shown to be benefit. I have attended many water and dry land births where the cord has not been felt for, and even when found the baby has been encouraged to deliver 'through' the cord without undermining the mother's ability to birth her baby. Handling and looping the cord over the head is a deep-seated 'skill' which midwives usually find incredibly difficult to change at a waterbirth (see Figure 7.5). My research has found books dating back as far as 1908 (Longridge) and 1914 (Andrews) explaining this method of dealing with the nuchal cord. It is unsurprising, therefore, that this is so difficult for midwives to move away from when it has been part of our practice for at least a hundred years!

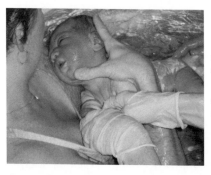

- Deliver baby's head
- Check cord patency and if intact deliver baby's body
- Allow baby to unravel in water
- Be patient

Figure 7.5   Cord entanglement

In a study published in 2007, Sadan et al. undertook a randomized controlled trial to assess neonatal outcomes (pH and Apgar score at 5 minutes) between two groups of nuchal cord babies. One group had the cord left intact whilst the other group had a pre-diagnosed nuchal cord (diagnosed during active labour using ultrasound) clamped and cut. The group who had the cord left intact either had it slipped over the head (if loose) or left (if too tight). The results of this study (albeit small – only 60 births in total) showed no adverse perinatal outcomes when either leaving the cord intact or cutting it. However, if as a midwife you have ever clamped and cut a cord and then had the problem compounded by shoulder dystocia (not in the water, I hasten to add), you will be as reticent as myself in never actively clamping or cutting the cord if it is around the baby's neck.

Anderson (2000) wrote that simple measures can assist the midwife with dealing with cord problems:

- Ensure the water is not unnecessarily deep – may occur as water is topped up during labour.
- Allow a little water to empty out as birth approaches back to level with breasts if it's overfilled.
- Have cord clamps ready for clamping cord if too short to bring baby to mother's arms – never clamp and cut underwater.
- Ensure baby is brought gently to the surface, being aware of undue tension to resistance in the cord – *remember baby may be unwrapped gently from cord under water with minimal touch or tension on cord* [my italics].
- Although cord snap is rare it is possible and should be at the back of your mind when delivering.

Cord snapping

Cro and Preston (2002) reported on four snapped cords (three where there were no adverse outcomes and one baby who needed resuscitation and blood transfusion – follow-up showed normal development) and highlighted the need for midwives to be prepared for this emergency. Two of the cases reported in this article were found to have normal-length cords and no excessive traction was placed upon the cord at delivery – hence the importance of ensuring cord patency prior to bringing the baby's whole body out of the water.

Interestingly, there was an ongoing debate in *Pediatrics* journal (2005) when the editorship was questioned regarding what was seen as a biased opinion against waterbirth. This ongoing issue of informed choice, knowledge and debate is important, but like Sheila Kitzinger I agree that it must be unbiased – we are all entitled to our own opinion but this must be balanced by evidence (both research and anecdotal, which is often more valued by midwives than doctors). The debate also raised the issue of cord snapping as a danger to the baby with water-birth. As described, the cord can be managed safely and efficiently if required.

Fetal hyperthermia

The question of a baby overheating *in utero* is one which is often asked when I teach. It would appear that whilst *in utero* the baby is reliant on its mother for controlling its temperature. A small rise in maternal temperature of 1 °C is thought to be highly unlikely to cause compromise. However, above that level – and certainly when a mother's temperature reaches 39 °C – the baby's temperature is thought to be 1 °C above its mother's. At higher temperatures the fetus has increased metabolic rate and oxygen demands (Charles 1998).

We are aware that newborns are susceptible at a temperature of 40 °C and may develop neonatal febrile convulsions. In the UK in 1993 two babies were delivered following a rise in maternal temperature and tachycardia (with resultant fetal tachycardia). It was when this tachycardia was heard that the mothers left the water and delivered on dry land. Both babies were born compromised. On reflection and discussion it transpired that the mothers' water and room temperatures were not clearly documented. Limited fluids were offered in the pool, change in maternal position was not encouraged and no guidance was given as to time in pool. It was unfortunate that this occurred in 1993 when other units surveyed revealed they had guidance in all these areas. It thus becomes important that we review guidelines for best practice, reflect on adverse outcomes and support education for midwives and parents.

Newborn inhalation of water

Hyponatremia at birth may occur as a result of swallowing fresh water. The fluid is absorbed quickly through the lungs into the circulation, which results in intravascular dilution and fluid overload. It has been suggested that if salt were added to pools the solution would be more isotonic, which would probably prevent the dilution and hyponatremia.

The problem with the issue above is that the newborn will not inhale because of the patent chemoreceptors which protect the baby's airway. If the physiology is understood – and thus when it is no longer safe to remain in the water – then inhalation will not occur. Where there have been 'drownings' this physiology has not protected the baby and a compromise has occurred. It is important therefore to investigate the change in physiology, and not just ban waterbirths. If a similar situation occurred with epidurals (low blood pressure causing fetal heart rate changes, even leading to assisted delivery), would we ban them?

Research Relevant to Practice

Eldering and Selke (1999), in 'Waterbirth in the 21st century', say that fetal breathing movements were initially demonstrated in 1974 by Dawes, who showed that babies do have rhythmic breathing *in utero*.

We do not believe that the lung fluid is squeezed out during birth but is absorbed over a period of hours. When asphyxia occurs, other overriding conditions also occur, which may cause premature fluid absorption and increased breathing activity, leading to aspiration. This may be a rationale for some of the adverse outcomes that have been documented.

Delayed cord clamping

Consensus of opinion about the timing of clamping the cord is difficult to obtain. Placental transfusion to the baby of 20–50 per cent of neonatal blood may be altered by the timing of when the cord is clamped, positioning of the baby in relation to gravity flow, and whether an oxytocic drug is used. The two sides of the argument cannot agree on the issue of transfusion to the newborn with associated hyperbilirubinaemia (due to increased red blood cells) There is also concern regarding respiratory distress resulting in an excess of plasma volume. Some babies will certainly not benefit from delayed cord clamping, rhesus isoimmunization being the obvious example. Interestingly, the World Health Organization (WHO 1996) recommends late cord clamping.

Neonatal polycythaemia

An article by Austin et al. (1997) is of interest since it is one of very few that has ever raised the issue of polycythaemia in the newborn. As there is delayed clamping and cutting of the cord with physiological third stage (or not at all if lotus birth occurs), there will be an associated high PCV (packed cell volume) and plasma viscosity. The umbilical cord should constrict on contact with air, but if the cord remains in warm water for a prolonged period the cord may well pulsate for longer, with the theoretical risk of polycythaemia. In Chapter 9 we will review many studies where this has not been identified as a problem.

In light of this one article I do not know of any practitioner who has altered their management of neonatal polycythaemia.

Questions for Discussion and Reflection

- Review your knowledge base on initiation of first breath and reflect on the differences with a waterbirth.
- Ask your colleagues to estimate one minute without looking at their watches. How accurate were they, and what are the implications of this for a waterbirth?

8
Interprofessional Issues in Waterbirth

This chapter will identify those other practitioners who may be able to assist midwives in planning, designing and implementing waterbirths. Where these people/departments have been involved, waterbirths appear to go from strength to strength. Throughout the world it seems that the amount of input from others varies depending on where and how we work. If anyone with a vested interested is included the service tends to be very positive, and it should be remembered that in some care settings non-involvement can result in poor outcomes. Infection control colleagues can assist in practical terms and auditing of any infection is an important issue of practice. Colleagues involved in moving and handling will be able to help with emergency evacuation – and also the basics, such as advising the midwife how to protect her back. Involvement of the supervisor of midwives and clinical governance departments will also be addressed.

Supervisor of Midwives

As discussed in Chapter 1, the role of the supervisor of midwives is enshrined in statute within the UK. Supervisors are involved in supporting the midwife and they act as an advocate for women, providing unbiased informed choice and discussion about options for care. They have an invaluable role to play in supporting midwives to identify learning needs, access educational requirements and guide them to reflect on their practice.

For mothers, they are often involved when women are seeking options for care, not just waterbirth – particularly when outside 'normal criteria'. It is vital that women know about supervisors and their role. The supervisor may assist in challenging and changing local guidelines, or help in finding other carers or independent midwives.

Infection Control

Specific use of infection control specialists will assist midwives who are supporting mothers with infectious illnesses. The most recent issues have been HIV-positive mothers with low viral loads who have been advised that they can have a vaginal birth. Enlightened practitioners are supporting mothers with a total non-touch technique. Specialists will be able to help with safety issues regarding protection of midwives (long gloves, non-touch technique), cleaning protocol (perhaps suggesting pools with liners) and cross-infection issues.

Any equipment that has contact with water needs to be sterilizable or disposable (although the latter is regarded as too expensive). The equipment, including the pool, needs to have appropriate cleaning protocols designed by infection control officers in collaboration with the pool company. However, as cited by Kitzinger (2005), the government enquiry by the expert advisory group on AIDS concluded that 'There is no evidence that HIV is any more likely to be transmitted from mother to a baby in a birthing pool than during birth elsewhere.'

Cleaning of pools and equipment should be performed using a chlorine-releasing agent, which is effective against HIV and hepatitis B and C.

Some units encourage mothers to bring in their own equipment (such as floatation aids/sieves). With a strict policy in place involving those people likely to clean the pool (cleaners, nurses, support workers or midwives), the risk of cross-infection is minimal. This is supported by the research outlined in Chapter 9.

Although midwives are advised to use a non-touch technique, there may be times when we need to place our hands in the water. We should have access to gauntlet gloves or sleeves; in reality, even if we wear gloves half a size smaller water is likely to seep into them. Whether this is an issue for practitioners depends on risk factors, and personal and professional responsibility.

Despite numerous studies (see Chapter 9) that show there is no increase in infection following bathing in water, many countries still do not encourage this practice once the waters have gone (amniotic fluid). Indeed, my American colleague Barbara Harper wrote about this issue in 2005, stating that many US hospitals do not support the use of water due to risk of ascending contamination infection. She quotes a 1960 article by Siegel, whose study proved this was impossible. He hoped his study would put to rest this misunderstanding and allow mothers to use water once their waters had gone. Sadly, as Barbara and I have both found around the world this is not the case. Box 8.1 lists the basic general principles for infection control in birthing pools.

Research Relevant to Practice

Hawkins (1995)
This was a study of 32 women, 16 water, 16 land – pre- and post-delivery screening:

- More micro-organisms were found in waterbirth than in land birth: 15:10
- None of the babies showed clinical signs of infection
- Colonization by *Staphylococcus aureus* was found, and in one case, E. coli

Comment: Cleaning policy – pipes. Normal colonization of bacteria in a birth environment.

Nyman (1999)
This was a study of 200 women, 100 waterbirths, 100 land.

- No increased infection rates were found in the two groups.
- Ruptured membranes < 24 hours
- Low risk

Comment: Intervention times for ruptured membranes and possible exclusions.

Comment: Infection is often a question raised with waterbirths. These small studies appear to show that it should not be of concern with appropriate risk assessment, cleaning policies and audit.

Fehervary et al. in 2004 wrote about a small study which highlighted one of the main concerns expressed about waterbirth. Infection is often cited as a reason not to use water, and as recently as 2008 this exact reason was given to a mother I met in Croatia. Her obstetrician had given all the other negative reasons for not using water and, finally, suggested that infection could be a risk. In all my clinical experience I

> **Box 8.1   General principles for infection control in birthing pools**
>
> - Use universal precautions for all mothers
> - Assess risk locally – HIV and hepatitis screening
> - Involve infection control department in planning
> - Utilize cleaning recommendations of pool manufacturers
> - Clean and dry pools pre- and post-use – part of daily domestic services
> - Do not use pool rooms as general storage areas
> - Ensure all equipment in contact with water is disposable or sterilizable
> - Carry out audit to establish whether you have an infection-free environment.

have never known of any infection in mother, newborn or midwife – indeed many specialists believe that in water any contamination is less infectious due to the amount of actual water. However, Fehervary's study of 96 mothers took microbiological swabs to identify faecal bacteria or environmental microbes from waterbirth and from conventional bed births with or without a relaxing bath. In all three groups they isolated most frequently from ear and palate of the newborns staphyloccus, E. coli and enterococci, which belongs to the normal vaginal flora. The rates of neonatal, infant and maternal infections did not differ between the three groups.

Moving and Handling

It is our own professional responsibility to protect our backs in whatever care settings we are working within. Water pools may place particular challenges on us, e.g., examination in water, pool cleaning (remember also to involve whoever will be cleaning the pools). We may lean over the pool when auscultating a fetal heart, performing a vaginal examination, assisting the baby to the surface, emergency situations; in all these circumstances we need to ensure minimal handling and stretching over the pool.

It is often assumed in midwifery that we have very few moving and handling issues. Personal correspondence from an M&H (moving and handling) trainer identified that midwives are notoriously bad at attending their mandatory training. However, when questioned, midwives did feel it was important, but admitted that other sessions (CTG, epidurals, breast feeding) had more relevance to their day-to-day work. With the introduction of birthing pools it has become vital that midwives not only attend manual handling sessions, and review current low-risk practices (alternative birth positions) and high-risk practice (equipment moving and mothers with epidurals), but also have good quality input regarding several issues surrounding the use of birthing pools. It is said that even bathing a baby when it is held away from the body and bending places a strain on the midwife's spine (Amos 2005). Using birthing pools for labour and delivery can place extra burden on midwives if this 'risk' is not assessed prior to the birth. This can include risk managers, supervisors of midwives and of course the clinical staff who will actually be using and cleaning the pool.

It is essential that we avoid twisting, and we should ensure that we bend from the knees and keep any carried loads close to our bodies.

The following are some general issues to consider for clinical practice:

- attend teaching sessions
- do a 'dry run'
- practise carrying equipment and setting up pools
- consider placement of pools – access to all sides is the ideal though not always practical
- have equipment within easy reach
- practise carrying out procedures such as ARM, VE and fetal heart auscultation
- use system of non-guarding of perineum and non-touch delivery including feeling for cord (this links with newborn physiology of first breath and reviewing the mechanism of labour – normal time frame for restitution of fetal head)
- assess risk for mothers with mobility problems
- assist mother in/out of pool
- watch out for water spillage.

Using the birthing pool

Ensure the following:

- posture: use cushions/birth balls/stools
- equipment: is it all to hand?
- minimum leaning over the pool
- setting up the pool: check pumps and pipes
- cleaning: ensure long-handed brush, shower
- emergency evacuation: know your skills drill.

Emergency evacuation for birthing pools

This is the procedure for emergency evacuation:

- call for assistance
- place floatation aids over the mother's head/arms/legs (see Fig 6.6)
- start to fill the pool to the top
- position a bed alongside the pool – same height as the lip of the pool
- position a pat board or slide mat at the edge of the bed/pool – apply brake
- place 'fishing net' under mother – ensure her head is supported by the top of the net (again see Fig 6.6)
- using water buoyancy, 'bounce' mother and lift to pat slide
- ensure good back posture and clear communication at all times
- continue to slide mother to top of bed – cover and dry her
- clear up any water spillages.

This procedure can be undertaken by three people – midwife, student/HCA and partner (although I suggest he only lifts the mother's legs).

This stepped procedure needs to be practised in any setting where a pool may be used (in a hospital or birth centre, emergency evacuation using this technique is often built into yearly skills drills). At home, midwives should have had the opportunity to practise this or at least ensure that those people present at the birth understand these principles and responsibilities.

A useful mnemonic, which I have adapted from Amos (2005), is:

E – equipment space (constraints, moving equipment around)
L – loads (unstable, bulky)
I – individual capability (midwives and mothers)
T – task to be achieved (examination with mother kneeling over edge of pool)
I – individual risk assessment (managers)
S – supports (appropriate moving equipment, evacuation procedures, skills drill)
T – training (attending sessions – general and specific)

Risk Management

A Health Service Executive (HSE) risk assessment and identification on the risk register is important to fulfil Trust requirements for safety. Most units in the UK have assessment undertaken during initial installation of a pool. It should include issues of spillages and pool leakage (rare). Estates departments will be able to assist midwives in planning issues such as protecting electrical plug sockets. Having toured numerous units throughout the world, I have been surprised by the difference in attitudes regarding water and electric sockets. In some units no electrical sockets are permitted; in others there are normal sockets; and others have covered electrical sockets. I do not believe it is our role as midwives to assess this risk; it will suffice simply to identify that electrical sockets may be required in or near the pool room, and then allow estates departments to organize the solution.

In a home situation, I always suggest that midwives discuss with parents the issues of water and electricity in close proximity, advising them to purchase childproof covers for any room sockets. These have three functions: there is less likelihood of plugging in electrical items whilst the pool is in use; water moisture is prevented from entering the socket; and, finally, parents will need to think through how they can use the CD player!

There maybe issues with hot water taps. In the UK there are COSHH (control of substances hazardous to health) regulations which place a limit to how hot the water can be in a birth centre or hospital. These can be negotiated if the importance of being able to quickly heat up the pool for delivery, and its inherent physiology, is explained to the engineers. At home this should not be an issue; we just need to be careful with children/animals and very hot water. What tends to be a problem at home waterbirths is the capacity of the hot water tank in relation to the size of the pool. It may be that the pool will take at least two tanks to fill; therefore the time it takes needs to be taken into account in planning a home waterbirth.

Engineers in hospitals and birth centres should be able to assist with planning appropriate heating, lighting and ventilation. In my experience they are very pleased to be involved, and when given the problem they have been able to arrive at a solution.

Finally, engineers can maintain standards of water cleanliness. Whilst most water supplies are clean and of a high standard in the UK, this may not be the case in all countries. If there is water contamination, it will mostly be by bacteria that are the mother's own; the contamination will be non-pathogenic and pose no risk to the baby. However, there are several situations that require further investigation, such as Legionnaires' disease and pseudomonas contamination.

Clinical Governance

NICE (2007) writes that clinical governance should be utilized in all clinical settings: multi-professional working, maintaining experience of staff rotating between obstetric and midwife-led units, clear referral pathways, use of supervisors of midwives with mothers who have risk factors, audit of practice and detailed root-cause analysis.

It may be unfair to place any issues surrounding litigation within the setting of clinical governance, but as part of the seven pillars of risk management it seems to be the most obvious place.

We cannot work within midwifery today without being aware that our society is becoming more litigious. Financial aid and the expert's role have changed over the past few years – particularly in the UK due to some high-profile cases – and there is now a new era of supportive expert work between all professionals involved.

The seven pillars of governance (shown in Box 8.2) can sit very comfortably with waterbirth services. I have added in italics my own thoughts on governance.

Box 8.2   The seven pillars of governance

Learning – *practical up-to-date education; multi-professional; wide-ranging and diverse subjects, e.g., physiological third stage*
Clinical effectiveness – *audit, i.e., quality and quantity issues*
Public experience – *surveys, audit, classes – unbiased information*
Strategic effectiveness – *governmental and local strategic support*
Resource effectiveness – *information to support care, IT and commerce*
Risk management – *link to CNST (Clinical Negligence Scheme for Trusts), health and safety, reporting adverse outcomes*
Communication – *a clear and safe message, guidelines and international awareness*

Setting Up a Waterbirth Service

There are plenty of references which offer the pros and cons in all issues of waterbirth. I would suggest that you review professional and consumer journals and utilize the references within this book.

Funding – initial and ongoing

Initial start-up costs may include the price of a pool, room changes, other equipment (net, hoist, underwater Doppler), education. Ongoing costs could include equipment and liners. These should all be estimated so that they can be included in any business plan. If you wish to be creative, consider buying home pools and 'hire' them out to mothers.

Suitable room

At home, advise parents about positioning their pool, ensuring as much access as possible. It should be near to plumbing. Ventilation and floor surfaces also need to be taken into consideration.

In hospitals and birth centres, ensure you are involved in initial planning to ensure the same factors as home births, but be aware that the room maybe multi-functional and you may need to gain access in an emergency.

Pool types

There are many pools now available – portable or plumbed in, specifically designed or adapted pools. Whichever you choose, if possible choose the largest that will fit into the room. You can make a pool smaller with flotation aids, but once it is installed you cannot make it any bigger! When we first designed the 'lagoon' pool, a pregnant midwife acted as our model, helping with size, depth, handles and angle of the sides.

Water availability

In most countries access to a readily available clean supply of water is not a problem. As already highlighted, the most common problem is with regard to home waterbirths and the size of domestic water boilers – these hold 40–60 gallons, whilst a pool may hold over 100 gallons. If there is inadequate hot water, the pool can be filled with the contents of one tank, then covered with a thermal cover (bubble wrap works very well) until a second tank's worth of hot water is available to top it up. I have known one incident where a new water filtration system was added to make the water clean; and heard that in Delhi, India, they were using bottled drinking water to fill the pool!

Guidelines for clinical practice

These should be written prior to starting your service. They need to reflect your care setting (home, birth centre or hospital), client groups and robust clinical care. They could also include any education issues or emergencies and multi-professional working (see Chapter 3).

Involvement of a multi-professional team

When planning a service you will find that many professionals will need to be involved (see above). However, it is important to remember that other practitioners who may influence or provide care to mothers (such as physiotherapists, complementary therapists, health visitors and general practitioners) can also have a profound effect. If you involve them and inform them of the waterbirth service and the evidence to support this option from the beginning, they will be more willing to embrace it.

Educational support

All practitioners involved with waterbirths are likely to require a degree of educational support. In Chapter 11 I have suggested some avenues for exploring various options, which midwives and other practitioners may wish to utilize.

Advertising to mothers

Ensuring that parents are aware of the pool service may be a delicate balancing act. Classes, aquanatal swimming and use of the media may all help to inform parents that a waterbirth service is available, but this must be balanced by not stressing water over other forms of analgesia, nor letting women have unrealistic expectations (bearing in mind there may be only one pool and limited midwives ready to support mothers).

Auditing and publishing

The sharing of experiences and audits is invaluable, as are presentations at local level – and, if possible, national and international level. Publish your findings at all levels; start with local papers, Trust newsletters and the local media; then, when ready, national or international journals.

Research Relevant to Practice

Cole (2004) surveyed birth centres in the USA and Canada to gain knowledge of practices in 72 centres. She obtained a 42 per cent response rate and a follow-up survey response rate of 62 per cent. She asked questions regarding pool types, informed consent, marketing the service, criteria for use and training for staff.

Conclusions: the majority of birth centres offered waterbirth. Midwives responded positively about their experiences. There were no neonatal or maternal deaths (total 10,132 births). Fifty-one per cent identified lower perineal trauma in waterbirth mothers. Problems were only reported by five units and included infection and shoulder dystocia.

Comments: The study identifies the need to share experiences and utilize skills and experiences of colleagues. It also identifies the response rate of postal surveys, Cole's rates being good at 42–62 per cent.

Costs of other forms of analgesia compared to water

There are several main issues regarding water versus other forms of analgesia. Firstly, the issue of choice and availability (ideas for challenging availability and criteria are given in Chapter 3). Secondly, the benefits of water as a non-invasive and non-interventionist form of analgesia (see Chapter 9). Thirdly, cost, which may have very different values depending on where and how you work. If total costs are required to be passed to the client or insurer (not something that mothers who use NHS services in the UK have to worry about) then cost effectiveness becomes more important.

Some of the costs are listed below (they are correct at the time of going to press).

Birthing pool
Cost: £150–£10,000
Water costs: £1.082 per 1000 litres of water (average pool holds 500–750 litres)

Birthing balls/chairs
Cost: £25–£2,500
Benefit: Mother can remain mobile and upright. Non-invasive and non-pharmacology analgesia.

TENS (transcutaneous electrical nerve stimulator)
Cost: hire £25, purchase £40–£70
Benefit: The mother remains in control of this analgesia; she is aware of her surroundings, can remain mobile and is drug free. May be used in all care settings where she can hire or purchase. Can be used with other forms of analgesia. See Melzack and Wall (1965).

Entonox (50% nitrous oxide and 50% oxygen)
Cost: 700 l cylinder gas £18.96
Low solubility inhalation analgesia. Utilized through the lung and arterial blood stream. Only small amounts required to saturate blood, thus high levels of arterial and brain tension of drug. Need to start as early as contraction felt – therefore there's a timing issue. Can be used with mask or mouthpiece; apparatus self-administered. High usage in UK, Australia and New Zealand.

Meptazinol
Cost: £1.92 per standard dose
Non-narcotic intra-muscular analgesia, used for the treatment of moderate to severe pain. Few side effects have been reported. May cause nausea/drowsiness and dizziness. Mild effects on fetus.

Narcotics
Cost: Pethidine 56p; Diamorphine £1.77; Demoral $1–2 per standard dose
Acts on opiate receptors at the neurone, causing analgesia, euphoria, sedation and possibly respiratory depression. May cause nausea and can cross over to the fetus. Timing of drug administration is important.

Anti-emetics
Cost: Maxolon 27p; Stemitil 54p; Cyclizine 49p per standard dose

Epidural
Cost: Fentanyl/Bupvicaine, pre-mixed bags £8
Epidural block acts on small-diameter autonomic nerve fibres. Advantages include long duration use, generally total analgesia and may allow mother to rest/sleep. May change nature of labour due to continuous monitoring, maternal position and changes to blood pressure (which may compromise fetus). Some older reports (MacArthur et al. 1990; Butler and Fuller 1998) showed that mothers suffer long-term sequelae with backache. However, more recent work (Howell et al. 2002

and Cochrane review, Cluett and Burns 2009) shows no significant increase in long-term backache.

And finally, many land births, particularly if pharmacological analgesia is given, require active management. The cost of Syntometrine (5 units oxytocin and 500 μg of Ergometrine) is £1.30, and Ergometrine 500 μg on its own is £1 per ampoule.

Questions for Discussion and Reflection

- Do you have specific moving and handling sessions for using your birthing pool?
- Have you considered all 'stakeholders' who may have a vested interest in the waterbirth service? Have you engaged with them?

9

Research

For me, the issue of research is linked to accountability: as practitioners we must ensure that our practice is evidence based. In the early years of waterbirth this was difficult; we were all just starting and there were no data available. However, this situation has changed dramatically over the past few years. Since the last edition of my book in 2000 there has been a plethora of published work. Why? Well, because many units were undertaking small numbers of waterbirths and needed to join together to have large enough numbers for any statistical analysis (Garland 2006a). Another reason was that larger units were themselves waiting until they had 2000 births to analyse before they felt able to publish. We now have large numbers in data sets from which two easy conclusions can be made. Firstly, it appears that most units have not been promoting waterbirth as better than land birth (although when you review the data you will see the results are better). The second conclusion is that no matter which country you work in, the results for waterbirths are very similar.

This chapter on research is vital to enable us as practitioners to have a balanced viewpoint of waterbirths, thus allowing us to provide accurate information to parents and ensure that we have a practice research bond.

McCraw (1989) wrote:

Throughout the struggles over [these] innovations in childbirth proponents have all too often made broad, sweeping and unsupported claims about the lasting benefits of these changes: similarly, opponents have frequently predicted dire calamities, also with limited supporting evidence, if such innovations are adopted. Advocates of the status quo have both the power of tradition and the weight of inertia on their side; it thus behooves proponents of changes to demonstrate that their innovations are both safe and beneficial. It is naïve to assume that mere anecdotal evidence or assertions that their innovation is 'more natural' will lead to its adoption by a medical profession that prides itself on its objectivity and scientific method.

The World Health Organization identifies that only 10 per cent of obstetrical procedures have been researched satisfactorily. Those of us supporting and introducing any new procedure need to ensure that it is adequately evaluated. One notable problem with the waterbirth data is that in many situations it is not possible to undertake a meta-analysis as the collected information is not always the same. Something as simple as an Apgar score is recorded as 'compromised' at different levels (Davidson 2002, Apgar < 5 at 1 minute; Geissbuehler et al. 2004, < 7 at 5 minutes; Garland 2006a, < 7 at 1 minute).

The data reproduced here are to highlight the information available and include a short comment on a personal level from myself. However, to start with I would like to consider what research we may need to consider when introducing and supporting waterbirth. Ideas of what may be required either as midwives or from our employer will be discussed. National and international research, including expanding parameters of research boundaries, will be included. Finally, the newest and most challenging research from around the world will be discussed with particular relevance to midwifery practice.

Audit

Audit is of value to all professionals and a simple sample audit form is reproduced in Figure 9.1. I would suggest that this is copied onto a double-sided sheet, which means midwives or mothers can add their comments easily. It is essential that you find a way of ensuring that the forms are returned to you and do not get lost. It is also useful to complete a form after a mother has been in the water for an hour, whether she stays in and delivers under water or not. This will give you data about which mothers leave the water and why, including further analgesia requirements and delivery outcomes. When this topic was locally audited by me in 1998, I found that there were three main reasons for leaving the water: further analgesia, fetal compromise or non-progress in labour. Utilizing the theories concept described in Chapter 4, we were able to reduce by half the number of mothers who left the water for further analgesia.

WATER LABOUR/BIRTH AUDIT FORM

Date:

Mother's demographic details:

Gravida: **Parity:**

Special considerations: (VBAC, GBS, other)

Dilation on entering water: .... cm (if recorded)

Duration of labour:

First stage timed from .... hours

Second stage timed from .... hours

Third stage timed from .... hours

Duration of immersion:

Entered water at .... hours

Left water at .... hours

Reason for leaving water: .... (third stage, slow labour etc.)

Outcome of delivery: .... (water, dry land, ventouse, LSCS)

Third stage management: dry land ☐   water ☐

Oxytocic given: No ☐   Yes ☐ Say what type: ....

Blood loss: < 500 ml ☐   > 500 ml ☐

Perineum: ....

Apgar score: At 1 minute: .... At 5 minutes: ....

Resuscitation required: ....

Baby to SCBU: No ☐   Yes ☐ State reason:............................

....

Method of feeding: breast ☐   formula ☐

Did mother attend any of the following classes?

aquanatal ☐   parent education ☐   general/specific ☐

Did mother make use of the following? internet ☐   leaflets ☐

Parents' comments: ....

....

....

....

Midwife's comments: ....

....

....

....

Figure 9.1   Sample water labour/birth audit form

Transferring audit data to a database

This is a simple format using a DOS edit program which can then be used with Excel programs to analyse the data (see Figure 9.2 for an example). Codes may be required for indicating age group, ethnicity, analgesia, reason for leaving the water.

Here are some of the comments documented through audit forms from both parents and midwives and personally collected over a 3-year period.

Parents' comments:

- 'I enjoyed the waterbirth. It felt calm and relaxing and helped my pain. Definitely the best of my four births.'
- 'Very relaxing. My second waterbirth and the best.'
- 'Lovely!! And relaxing.'
- 'Perfect delivery. No problems. Lovely to have such great midwives.'
- 'Very happy and quick.'
- 'Nice relaxing delivery. It all happened so fast.'

	Water	Dry land
Parity		
Age group		
Ethnicity		
First stage		
Second stage		
Cervical dilation		
Analgesia		
Third stage management		
Estimated blood loss (EBL)		
Perineum		
Apgar scores		
TOS		
Home/birth centre/hospital		
Reason for leaving water		

Figure 9.2 Waterbirth audit – water versus dry land birth

- 'Calm and peaceful environment – thank you for all your support. First waterbirth in hospital – this one was at home in your pool – thank you.'
- 'So much calmer than my first delivery.'

Midwives' comments:

- 'A nice relaxing normal delivery.'
- 'Lovely and calm experience – husband's support was superb.'
- 'A wonderful relaxing time was had by all.'
- 'Interesting as mother had not planned to have a waterbirth – liked the water so much she did not want to get out.'
- 'Mother was empowered by the pool, she was very much in control and coped well with only water and entonox.'
- 'Very calm lovely delivery. Easy for mother to move around the pool.'
- 'My first ever waterbirth as a qualified midwife – saw two as a student – but this one was great.'
- 'Peaceful, calm and relaxing.'
- 'So relaxing – brilliant.'

Research and audit

There have been many claims made about the benefits of waterbirth (see some original advantages and disadvantages in Chapter 2). Over its history, Waterbirth International USA have made claims regarding the benefits of water. They say it:

- speeds up labour
- reduces blood pressure
- gives the mother greater feeling of control
- provides significant pain relief
- promotes relaxation
- enables the mother to assume any position which is comfortable for labour/birth
- conserves her energy
- reduces the need for drugs and interventions
- gives the mother a private protected space
- reduces perineal trauma and eliminates episiotomy
- reduces Caesarean section rates
- is highly rated by mothers – typically stating they would consider giving birth in water again

- is highly rated by experienced providers
- encourages an easier and gentler welcome for the baby.

Comment: Since much of this is anecdotal evidence from parents and practitioners, it is difficult to substantiate through research. That is not to say it is not of value, but in the evidence-based culture within which we work, some practitioners may wish for more robust information.

It may be difficult to seek research funding to establish or challenge some of these claims and this is often an issue for those practitioners wishing to further establish credibility for them. One of the concerns of midwives and medics alike regarding waterbirth has been the surrounding evidence upon which to base practice. Despite numerous studies, many of which are highlighted in this chapter, there are always issues concerning the fact that most are not randomized, controlled trials; many are audits and thus do not appear in systematic reviews and databases (i.e. Cochrane.) This in itself may say more about the editing and publication of a particular journal than about the evidence provided.

I am reproducing here some of the latest work that has been produced on waterbirth. However, many authors have been publishing data for many years, and this work should not be undervalued despite it being older information.

Pinette et al. (2004) wrote that although they recognized that many waterbirths had occurred, 'most of these accounts are retrospective and *uncontrolled* [my italics] and represent reports of individuals or institutional experiences'. Several issues need to be raised regarding this statement. Firstly, what other type of data does Pinette expect other than individual or institutional? Many authors have years of clinical experience and evidence, and some (such as Garland 2006a) was multicentred. As an author and practitioner who has studied waterbirths for many years, I feel the comment about their being uncontrolled is totally unjustified. Work that I have been involved in has been supported by a researcher and the hospital audit department; it has been presented and scrutinized through clinical governance and then published.

Pinette is right to raise the issue of adverse outcomes, which should be investigated, but he appears not to have reviewed the physiology of first breath with his comment about newborns taking a breath under water (see Chapter 7). He continues by stating that Cochrane could find no evidence that perineal trauma, duration of labour or use of analgesia is reduced. The data below may assist him in altering and reviewing his opinion. Finally, one may ask, as did an obstetrician in Portland, USA, how many waterbirths he has actually attended.

As far back as 2001 Stewart highlighted the differences in how professionals regard sources of data analysis. It appears that medical staff view the gold standard as randomized controlled trials, whilst midwives seem to also value experience, reflection, history and intuition. This basic difference in the various merits of research causes problems with assessment of waterbirths, since, as already stated, much data is anecdotal, qualitative, audit and of course personal experiences. Should we undervalue these other options? Much of this discussion is outside the remit of this book but I believe that experience should be as valued as much as pure research; the two balance our experiences and are often defined by where and how we work, and by colleague support and conflicts that we encounter. Stewart concludes by writing, 'health professionals may create a culture, intentionally or otherwise, which becomes a means of asserting a system of authoritative knowledge. The term evidence-based practice implies that it should be value free ... but this is far from true'.

When I started work with other units in 1999 to collect data from 10 units around the country (published 2002 and 2006) we had much debate about the relative merits of undertaking a randomized control trial (RCT). Most of the 10 units had been supporting waterbirths for many years, and women chose to give birth at the unit knowing that if all remained low risk they had a good chance of delivering in water. Would these women therefore be willing to enter a RCT and reduce this opportunity?

In debating this, many of the group thought women would not. However, one small pilot study by Woodward (2004) attempted to answer a fundamental question as to whether mothers would be willing to join an RCT. Northampton Hospital was part of the Garland (2004) audit and during this process, as already stated, much debate ensued between group participants regarding the various merits of audit versus RCT. The main argument against was that mothers had often spent time and energy in deciding on various options for labour and delivery (often even changing maternity units in order to find one which would support her choice of waterbirth) and would be unwilling on the day to be selected into a RCT. However, Woodward showed (albeit with a small group of mothers – 80 women, of whom 60 entered the trial), that it was possible to undertake an RCT.

Comment: I would ask, though, why 20 mothers (25 per cent) did not continue in the study. Was it because of the original debate – that having chosen water they wished to continue with it – or did complications arise? This study is small and to the best of my professional knowledge has not been repeated. Most data collection remains retrospective audit and personal experiences.

Summary of clinical audit outcomes

Box 9.1 lists authors who have written on the advantages and disadvantages of water. Some are their own clinical experiences and others are audits.

Box 9.1   Authors writing on advantages and disadvantages of water

Advantages

- Weightless
- Relaxing

Edlich et al. (1987);
Church (1989)

- Reduces muscle tension
- Reduces anxiety
- Reduces catecholamines
- Increases endorphins

Ginesi et al. (1998)

- Increases uterine perfusion
- Decreases pain contraction
- Produces shorter labour
- Reduces need for augmentation

Schorn et al. (1993)
Garland (2000a)
Geissbuehler et al. (2000)

- Increases elasticity of perineum
- Reduces tears
- Has effects on cardiovascular system

Burns (2001)
Alderdice et al. (1995)
Cefalo et al. (1978)

- Reduces blood pressure
- Increases maternal satisfaction
- Increases sense of control

Hall and Holloway (1998)
Richmond (2003)

Disadvantages

- Creates unrealistic expectations
- Restricts other analgesia choices
- Restricts mobility
- Reduces contraction effectiveness
- Increases perineal trauma

McCandlish and Renfrew
(1993)

- Increases risk of maternal vaginal infection
- Increases risk of injury to midwives' backs
- Relaxes uterine muscle = increased bleeding
- Increases risk of MROP
- Increases maternal temperature = increased neonatal temperature
- Allows possibility of water emboli
- Can be delay in emergency evacuation

Rosevear et al. (1993)
Alderdice (1995)
Church (1989)
Deans (1995)
Johnson (1996)
Deans (1995)
Odent (1983)
Zimmerman (1993)

Finally ...

Alderdice et al. (1995) undertook a review of 2885 women, and Gilbert and Tookey (1999) surveyed 4032 women. Both surveys indicated that there was no reliable evidence to justify denying the choice of water immersion for labour and or birth to women at low risk of complications.

Some Early Studies

The studies below show that waterbirth outcomes have been audited for many years, from 1987 when Lenstrup first published his small study showing no adverse outcomes, through to Garland (2006a). The studies vary greatly in size and are from various parts of the world but show that no matter where you work similar results are recorded. They indicate no major adverse outcomes for mother or baby (of course some mothers will have a third-degree tear or postpartum haemorrhage just as can occur on dry land) and results show, I believe, that in a skilled practitioner's care, water can offer a safe alternative for labour and birth.

Lenstrup et al. (1987)

Eighty-eight women bathed for between ½ hour and 2 hours during the first stage of labour. Higher rates of morphine use and oxytocin stimulation in non-bath group – not significant. No differences in operative delivery, perineal trauma, bleeding or neonatal condition. Duration of labour the same in both groups. Minimal water contamination – not significant and no significant febrile episodes postnatally.

Doniec-Ulman et al. (1987)

The study showed a decrease in blood pressure when women were immersed in water during labour – these changes did not appear to be related to changes in hormonal levels. The following were observed:

- decrease in respiration rate
- decrease in lactic acid levels
- decrease in O_2 consumption
- decrease in muscle tone
- decrease in cortical levels

- increase in perfusion to internal organs
- increase in skin temperature
- increase in electrical resistance of skin
- water needs to be deep enough to reduce gravity
- buoyancy – weightlessness; reduced pressure on vena cava
- less energy and oxygen expended to maintain body temperature
- adrenaline reduced
- emotional wellbeing increased.

Geissbuehler et al. (2000)

This is a study that was carried out in Switzerland between 1991 and 1997. There were 2014 births. Waterbirth was compared with bed delivery and birthing stool. Waterbirth showed the following benefits:

- lowest blood loss
- fewer painkillers
- increased birth experience
- higher Apgar scores and average arterial pH levels
- no higher neonatal infection than in other methods
- no water aspiration or other complications.

Otigbah et al. (2000)

This was a study of 301 births carried out at Rochford Hospital, Southend, UK, between 1989 and 1994. The results showed:

- primips (primiparae) had a shorter first stage, reduced analgesia requirements, less perineal trauma
- non-waterbirth group had twice as many third-degree tears, increased PPH rate (2.7% compared with 1.3%)
- one maternal pyrexia – no positive cultures
- two waterbirth babies were admitted to SCBU (one true knot in cord, one compound presentation)
- Apgars were comparable; no neonatal deaths.

Burns (2001)

This study reported on 2357 mothers between 1990 and 1998 – matched non-pool users by parity, spontaneous onset > 37/40 cephalic presentation, singleton pregnancy and uncomplicated pregnancy with no previous Caesarean section. There were 627 primips and 745 multips. Thirty-eight per cent of waterbirths used aromatherapy.

In water:

- a higher number of spontaneous vertex delivery (SVD)
- higher intact perineums.

SCBU admissions:

- water 1.2%
- dry land 2.5%.

Davidson (2002)

This was a study at the John Flynn Hospital, Australia, of 127 water-births over 3 years. Age range was 24–43 years (average 31). Parity: 53 primips; 74 multips. VBAC: 4.

These were the results:

- spontaneous delivery: 94; induced delivery: 33
- pool entry average dilation: 3–4 cm
- average length of time in pool: 132 minutes
- average length of labour of primigravida mothers:
    o first stage: 5 hours 58 min
    o second stage: 63 min
    o third stage:16 min
- average length of labour of multigravida mothers:
    o first stage: 4 hours 18 min
    o second stage: 15 min
    o third stage: 12 min
- 123 of 127 had active dry land third stage
- perineal trauma: 53 were intact (41%)
- complications: tender uterus (treated with antibiotics) – two
                postpartum haemorrhage – two
                manual removal of placenta – four
- Apgars: < 5 at 1 minute – five (3.9%)
          < 5 at 5 minutes – two needed O_2
- no third-degree trauma.

Thni and Mussner (2003)

This study was undertaken in Sterzing, South Tyrol, and compared 1500 births.

	Waterbirth	Land birth – bed	Birthing stool
Number	969	515	172
Average length first stage	381 minutes	473 minutes	
Second stage	No difference		
Episiotomy	0.52%	17.2%	7.6%
Perineal trauma	23% all groups		
Primips – intact perineum	58%	36%	48%

Comment: Other factors examined – arterial cord pH, maternal Hb (base and postnatal) – showed no difference. Waterbirth appears safe for mother and fetus/neonate if candidates are selected appropriately.

Geissbuehler et al. (2004)

This was a 9-year observational study carried out in Switzerland.

	Water	Land
Number	3617	5901
Primips	1238	
Multips	2379	
First stage (mean in minutes)	272.6	307
Second stage	26.2	36.2
Perineal trauma		
Intact	34.2%	29.2%
First/second-degree tear	50.1%	41.1%
Third/fourth-degree tear	2.3%	3.6%
Episiotomy	8.3%	25.7%
Maternal infections		
Fever > 38 °C	10	30
Neonatal outcomes		
pH	7.29	7.27
Apgar < 7 at 5 minutes	4	19
Apgar < 9 at 10 minutes	10	46
NICU admissions	6	37
Shoulder dystocia	6	16
Infection	20	60

Thoeni et al. (2005)

This study was carried out in Vipitena/Sterzing, Italy. It compared 1600 waterbirths at a single institution over an 8-year period between 1997 and 2004.

Maternal outcomes

	Water n = 737	Bed n = 407	Birthing stool n = 142	p-value
First stage (minutes)	380	468	*	< 0.01
Expulsion (minutes)	34	37	35	n.s.
Cord pH	7.27	7.26	7.24	n.s.
Base excess	−5.35	−6.09	−6.82	n.s.
Episiotomy	0.68%	23.3%	8.4%	< 0.01
First-degree tear	23.7%	22.3%	23%	n.s.
Second-degree tear	11.4%	11%	13%	n.s.
Third-degree tear	0.95%	0.9%	2.1%	n.s.
Day 1 Hb	10.9	10.1	10.23	n.s

Neonatal outcomes

	Waterbirth n = 986	Delivery on land n = 647
Clinical signs of infection	1.22% (n = 12)	2.63% (n =17)
C-reactive protein mg/dl	1.5–0.2	2.82–1.82
Arterial cord pH	7.25	7.24
Base excess	−5.35	−6.05
Birth weight (average, in grams)	3268 (2480–4660)	3245 (2090–4570)

A bacterial filter was introduced in 2002 after water samples showed high levels of *Pseudomonas aeruginosa* and *Legionella pneumophila* – interestingly, there was no increase in infection rates in the waterbirth group.

Garland (2006a)

This was a 2-year audit of clinical outcomes in 10 waterbirth care settings within the United Kingdom. All units had established waterbirth services, had clinical audit department support and agreed to meet during the audit to discuss clinical experiences and outcomes.

There were 2000 waterbirths with matched groups of mothers matched by age, parity, ethnicity, home or hospital and VBAC. The ratio of primigravid mothers to multigravid mothers was 50:50. (The ratio at birth centres was 30:70. This may have been in part to the criteria for using a birthing centre: in some situations this was limited to multi-gravid mothers.)

Cervical dilation varied between 1 cm to 10 cm, with a mean of 6 cm. This shows the variability of when mothers go into the pool. Sometimes this was suggested in the unit's guidelines (based on history, pool availability or time to unit). Most units in the study did not have a starting point and it was left to the midwife and mother to decide when was the appropriate time to enter the water.

For previous LSCS mothers, four of the study units offered VBAC in water. Whilst this only accounted for 0.7 per cent of the study group, there was no scar dehiscence. One unit offered formal risk assessment (see Chapter 3).

	Primips water	Primips land	Multips water	Multips land
Length of labour (mean in minutes)	351	423	219	260
Perineal trauma				
Intact	33.8%	18.2%	41.7%	33.6%
Third-degree tear	1.4%	1.5%	0.3%	0.9%
Overall rates for primips and multips	Water 14 (0.7%)	Land 18 (0.9%)		
PPH > 500 ml	3%	6.6%	4%	4%
Apgars < 7 at 1 minute	0.14%	0.7%	0.15%	0.53%
Overall rates for primips and multips	Water 3 (0.15%)	Land 12 (0.6%)		

Other studies

Eckert et al. (2001), Garland (2002), Gradert et al. (1987) and McCandlish et al. (1998) may also be mentioned. For other studies which may be useful, consult the Reference list and the Further Reading list at the end of this book.

'The gold standard' Cochrane review (2009)

This review was undertaken by Cluett and Burns, two authoritative midwives who have both practised waterbirth. *Immersion in Water in Labour and Birth* was a follow-up from a 2004 review (see Nikoderm, which was withdrawn) undertaken by Cochrane.

This paper highlights some of the government documents which have given some official acceptance to water immersion, and summarizes the effects on mothers and babies during its use. Unlike the last Cochrane review, it references audits that have been undertaken prior to the actual review of randomized control trials.

Nineteen studies were identified, which for the purpose of the review addressed 'outcomes on physical and psychological health and well-being'. As with many audits, similar data were analysed including issues of maternal morbidity (blood loss, infection, perineal trauma) and neonatal outcomes (Apgar at 5 minutes, infection, snapped cord). It is beyond the scope of this book to reproduce the full document but I will aim to summarize the review.

Maternal outcomes – immersion in first stage

	Result	*Studies reviewed*
Immersion in water in first stage	Reduced use of epidural	Cammu et al. (1994); Eckert et al. (2001); Kuusela et al. (1998); Ohlsson et al. (2001); Rush et al. (1996); Woodward (2004)
Use of narcotic/pethidine	No significant difference	Eckert et al. (2001); Rush et al. (1996); Taha (2000); Woodward (2004)
Mode of delivery	No significant difference	Cammu et al. (1994); Eckert et al. (2001); Kuusela et al. (1998); Ohlsson et al. (2001); Rush et al. (1996); Taha (2000); Woodward (2004)
Slowing of labour (analysed by use of amniotomy/oxytocin use)	No significant difference in amniotomy or oxytocin use	da Silva et al. (2007); Kuusela et al. (1998); Rush et al. (1996); Schorn et al. (1993)
Duration of first or second stage	No significant difference	Cammu et al. (1994); da Silva et al. (2007); Eckert et al. (2001); Kuusela et al. (1998); Rush et al. (1996); Schorn et al. (1993); Woodward (2004)

	Result	*Studies reviewed*
Perineal trauma	No significant differences in intact, tears or episiotomy rates	da Silva et al. (2007); Eckert et al. (2001); Ohlsson et al. (2001); Rush et al. (1996); Taha (2000) Woodward (2004)
Maternal infection	No significant difference	Cammu et al. (1994); Eckert et al. (2001); Kuusela et al. (1998); Rush et al. (1996); Schorn et al. (1993)
Maternal experience of pain	Reduced experience in water	Taha (2000)
Reduced blood pressure	Statistically significantly reduced	Taha (2000)

Comment: The data seem to suggest that there is no great significant difference in maternal outcomes for mothers who labour in water. The reviewers themselves have identified that some studies are very small (e.g., Taha 2000) and that even a simple analysis of length of labour can be hard due to varying interpretations of 'in labour'. Meta-analysis was therefore very difficult because of variables in the trials. This is especially true of studies when Apgar score is identified as 'compromise' at different scores or indeed at 1 or 5 minutes.

Neonatal outcomes – mothers immersed in first stage

	Result	*Studies reviewed*
Gestational age at birth	No difference	Cammu et al. (1994); da Silva et al. (2007); Eckert et al. (2001); Kuusela et al. (1998); Ohlsson et al. (2001); Rush et al. (1996); Schorn et al. (1993); Taha (2000); Woodward (2004)
Apgar < 7 at 5 minutes	No significant differences	Cammu et al. (1994); Eckert et al. (2001); Ohlsson et al. (2001); Schorn et al. (1993); Taha (2000)

	Result	Studies reviewed
Mean Apgar at 5 minutes	No difference	da Silva et al. (2007); Rush et al. (1996)
Admissions to NICU	No significant difference	Eckert et al. (2001); Ohlsson et al. (2001); Woodward (2004)
Infection rates	Vey low	Cammu et al. (1994); Eckert et al. (2001); Kuusela et al. (1998); Rush et al. (1996); Schorn et al. (1993)

Comment: Neonatal outcomes for mothers who have laboured (but not delivered) in water show no significant differences from dry land birth. It is interesting that the trials have decided upon an Apgar of less than 7 at 5 minutes as a marker of compromised neonate. This caused considerable debate in the Garland audit (2006a) and may be an improved method of assessing compromise; it excludes the first breath 'blue baby' issue which is seen with waterbirths (see Chapter 7).

Maternal outcomes – immersion in second stage

	Result	Studies reviewed
Mode of delivery	No significant difference	Nikoderm et al. (1999); Woodward (2004)
Perineal trauma	No significant difference	Nikoderm et al. (1999); Woodward (2004)
Birth experience	Better birth experience in water	Nikoderm et al. (1999)

Comment: These are important data, although the results of only a few studies, to support midwives who wish to offer this choice of birth. The birth experience issue has been addressed in some audits (see below) but does need further investigation. There are compounding factors which include one-to-one care, supportive midwives and an understanding and belief in physiological labour.

Neonatal outcomes – mothers immersed in second stage

	Results	Studies reviewed
Incidence of meconium	No significant difference	Nikoderm et al. (1999); Woodward (2004)
NICU admissions	No significant difference	Nikoderm et al. (1999); Woodward (2004)
Low Apgars	No significant difference	Nikoderm et al. (1999); Woodward (2004)
Arterial pH	No significant difference	Nikoderm et al. (1999); Woodward (2004)
Raised neonatal temperature > 37.5 °C	No significant difference	Nikoderm et al. (1999)

Comment: Despite the fact that concern is often expressed that babies will 'drown' or have infections, there have actually been very few data collected on neonatal outcomes. Some data do exist in audits but it would appear that this is an area that requires further investigation.

Early versus late immersion in water

	Result	Studies reviewed
Early versus late immersion	Significant increase in epidurals and augmentation with early immersion	Ericksson et al. (1997)

Comment: This is an interesting aspect of care. There has often been debate about when is the 'right' time for a mother to enter the water. Although an early study, this factor should be considered in clinical practice, and is further raised in Chapter 5.

Caregiver outcomes: No trial describes any injuries or satisfaction outcomes for caregivers.

Third stage of labour: The reviewers are not aware of any RCTs regarding third stage management. The issue of water emboli is highlighted in Odent (1983) and challenged by Wickham (2003).

The Newborn Perspective

There has been very little study done from the baby's perspective. That which has been undertaken tends to review clinical parameters (Apgar scores, cord pH, neonatal temperatures). The focus of whether water has any benefits to the newborn's development has been omitted.

In Smirnov (2002) the author summarized work from Russia based on Charkovsky's waterbabies, who stood early, understood speech symbols, did not exhibit aggressive behaviour and displayed telepathic and other extrasensory abilities. Smirnov's study followed children who took part in regular swimming from the first few days of life. Various parameters included physical growth and cognitive functions. He concluded that babies born in water develop faster than dry land babies. This study needs repeating and I believe would have more credibility in the UK if supported by an organization such as the Tavistock Institute.

In 1986 Ray wrote 'that with water training programmes these children ... are more confident, lack aggression, are more intelligent, rarely fall sick and easily withstand cold and weather changes ... they are said to have no temper tantrums, sleep soundly, are physically stronger, more active, brighter and resourceful'. To the best of my knowledge this work has never been substantiated and does little to add credence to waterbirth.

As a midwife I just want to ensure that the babies grow up healthy and happy; any other benefits are probably the result of a number of factors, including the mother's own perception of her birth experience.

Psychological Aspects of Water

Wu and Chung (2003)

This study identified several reasons why mothers chose water for labour and birth. These women lived in Taiwan, where water was a relatively new concept for birth, although it was certainly known to both parents and practitioners. There were several themes which appeared during this small study: (1) dissatisfaction with the current medical care system (women were encouraged to have LSCS) and perceived lack of respect, warmth, support or autonomy on the part of hospitals; (2) previous negative delivery experiences, 'negligence of medical staff'; (3) experience that falls short of expectations, a medical system that does not allow for birth companions, immediate breast feeding or VBAC support.

The next main issues are grouped together under 'demonstration of autonomy': women wish to choose their own childbirth methods, trust the midwife, fulfil their individual dignity, ensure consideration for their relatives/partners, and employ strategies to achieve these goals.

This was only a very small study (nine mothers) and therefore one must question how reflective this was of Taiwanese mothers generally. However, I have no reason to suspect that these mothers are alone in their thoughts about medical care in Taiwan; it may be that other mothers have not had the opportunity to express their concerns. The study needs to be repeated; unfortunately, I feel it reflects many other countries around the world.

Richmond (2003)

This study, which covered five birthing centres in the UK, wished to explore two main questions:

1. What are the experiences of women who have a waterbirth?
2. Do all women perceive waterbirth as therapeutic?

The study took a random sample of 240 women from 482 mothers who experienced a waterbirth in south-east England over a 2-year period.

Mothers' reasons for choosing waterbirth:
- 'Thought it seemed more natural' 78%
- 'Thought it would be less painful in water' 78%
- 'Thought it would be gentle delivery for the baby' 72.6%
- 'Wanted a drug-free labour' 50.3%
- 'Love warm water' 91%
- 'Thought it would prevent tearing' 37.6%
- 'Had it recommended' 27.4%
- 'Thought it would prevent interference from others' 24.2%
- Other reasons 17.7%

Mothers' feelings when entering the pool:
- 'Relaxation' mentioned 99 times
- 'Relief' mentioned 51 times
- 'Pain relief' referred to 50 times
- 'Warmth' was used 48 times

Other words used to describe their experiences: 'buoyancy', 'control' and 'calming'

Differences between waterbirth and previous birth experiences:
- 'More in control' 39 mothers
- 'More relaxing' 28 mothers
- 'Less painful' 24 mothers

Expanding Parameters

VBAC (vaginal birth after Caesarean) care has become a particular hot potato over the past few years, with mothers seeking alternatives to repeat LSCS (lower segment Caesarean section).

In 1998 I was in the privileged position of working within an enlightened environment which had a positive attitude to supporting mothers with low-risk assessment for midwifery care in labour. The confidence and support that was available has been described in various articles in the last few years. Mayer (2004) writes about her home birth VBAC experience with an independent midwife. She describes the appointments with registrars in her antenatal clinic who openly accused her of wanting a vaginal delivery 'more than a healthy baby'. It is appalling to me that any mother should have to hear this type of arrogant comment from a professional, whose own medical education would have not enabled him to view childbirth as normal. The empowering role that a midwife offers women is often stifled in the NHS and therefore many women choose an independent midwife to obtain their right to choice.

An empowering team at Maidstone Hospital in Kent designed a risk assessment tool. Garland (2006b) discussed this tool and examined the results of 92 mothers who between 2002 and 2004 undertook to use water after a previous LSCS. The results supported the multi-professional approach to selecting low-risk criteria for VBAC mothers who may use water. Clinical outcomes – mode of delivery, analgesia, birth weight and Apgar scores – were all recorded. One scar dehiscence occurred in a mother who had not used water and was detected following an abnormal admission CTG. The VBAC rate for mothers who had spontaneous onset was 87 per cent; induced was 66 per cent. Total VBAC rate for these mothers who were risk-assessed was 70 per cent, compared to 30 per cent for the mothers who chose not to proceed with the risk assessment process.

Mothers' VBAC rate was based on previous LSCS: elective (highest percentage was previous breech presentation, 33 per cent) 75 per cent; emergency (previous LSCS 61 per cent; 24 per cent failure to progress).

In summary, I believe this tool was invaluable in supporting mothers with choice. There is now an underwater CTG transducer which can be used to monitor VBAC mothers in water. This, combined with good skills in waterbirth and dry land low-risk VBAC care, could be used as guidance for the future care of VBAC mothers. In Garland (2004) I wrote that I believe the process of risk assessment in itself may reinforce the mother's belief in her own ability to give birth.

In 2004 Cluett et al. published a small study (99) of mothers who used water rather than traditional augmentation in labour dystocia (cervical dilation rate < 1 cm per hour in active labour). The traditional augmentation warranted amniotomy and intravenous oxytocin. Whilst some of the mothers who initially entered the water did eventually require traditional augmentation, the operative delivery rates were similar. Apgar scores, infection rates and cord pH showed no difference. This study needs repeating.

If practitioners wish to explore other aspects of research and waterbirth, I would recommend Redwood's (1999) review of discourse analysis of waterbirth texts. Whilst not a new paper, its approach to analysis is still of relevance and can assist in placing some of the aforementioned studies within a new context.

Suggested other areas for audit or research

The following areas would all benefit from audit/research:

- aquanatal preparation
- analgesia requirements
- cost effectiveness
- uptake patterns
- breast feeding rates
- maternal/newborn infection rates
- postnatal/child development
- subjective comments from parents
- midwives' comments and experiences
- SCBU admissions
- management of complications
- adverse outcomes.

In 2005 Keirse (a professor of obstetrics in Adelaide, Australia) wrote about conducting randomized control trials with waterbirth. He quotes from other studies that the recorded risk of complications is very low (including 'wet lung', which occurs with LSCS not just waterbirth). But is it really ethical to undertake an RCT to prove 'harm' to the newborn? 'If there is one thing on which the staunchest foes are unanimous, it is that the RCT is an ineffective tool to detect, let alone quantify, rare, but serious adverse effects of an intervention. If that were its purpose, few trial proposals would ever survive the scrutiny of an ethical committee.' He concludes:

> I am even more strongly biased in favour of RCT. Bias permits one to forego the one-way traffic from introduction, through methods and results, up to conclusions when reading a paper, and start with the last one or two sentences instead. When doing so, we learn that a RCT of water birth might reduce the average intelligence of mankind, while being definitely needed and eminently feasible. As there is nothing to substantiate either one of these opinions when reading back to front, we may as well stick to my bias and show RCT some respect by using it appropriately and for genuine inquiries instead of mere decoration.

This is a sentiment similar to that expressed by Garland and Jones (2000), when discussing why practice evaluation was audit and not research. 'We often considered changing to the clinical research approach but rejected this because we recognized a number of ethical and practical constraints.' We continued with audit because we had many ethical debates about withholding an analgesic which we had shown to be beneficial through numerous papers (1994 and 1997).

Conclusion

Although there are many data now available for practitioners to review, we cannot be complacent. It is vital that if waterbirth is new to your hospital, birth centre or practice that you audit and evaluate results. It is essential that you are able to provide quantitative and qualitative data from mothers and midwives. And, finally, this information needs to be shared with others both nationally and internationally.

I finish with another quote from McCraw (1989):

If waterbirth or any other innovation in childbirth proves anxiety reducing or otherwise more pleasurable for the couple and not dangerous to the foetus, that is enough and it should be available as an option. It is not necessary that it results in a new breed of human. Such scientifically unsupported claims leave one open to questions of honesty and ethics, if not litigation, in today's society. What should always be kept in mind, it seems to this writer, is freedom of choice. Replacing an inflexible system that does not allow waterbirth with one that would require every woman to labour and deliver in a tub of water is surely no improvement.

Questions for Discussion and Reflection

- Review your own local data collection. How does it compare with the national and international outcomes?
- What further audits would you like to commence?

10

Teaching and Ongoing Education

Ongoing education for midwives is vital to help us maintain credibility as practitioners. This chapter will explore ideas for education via sessions, websites, videos and resources. This will include local and national educational needs in line with UK professional education requirements. Included in this chapter will be a section on midwifery competences.

The issue of extra education and training arises in Miller and Magill-Cuerden (2006). Miller reminds us that as long ago as 1994 the UKCC (UK Central Council) identified waterbirth as normal midwifery practice. Why is it that we believe we need extra training? I have never believed that 'going to a lecture, watching three, doing three, then starting' should be adopted as the correct process; rather, I believe that midwives should decide for themselves when they have reached their own level of confidence and competence, and not be dictated by an arbitrary number. Many units now use waterbirth as an educational opportunity: see one, do one and then start.

Accountability and competence is important for all practitioners and education should include all staff including medical staff, support workers and students. All members of staff need to have up-to-date skills and knowledge.

Learning from Each Other

Stories from parents and professionals

These stories identify different experiences from healthcare practitioners and mothers who have experienced waterbirths in various settings worldwide. Read them, and then reflect on what can be learnt from each story and ponder any impact they may have on your practice.

Lindy – waterbaby, UK
When I was born I first saw mumma and dada and two other ladies, they were mummas midwives. The first thing I did was scream and cry in mamas arms I soon calmed down a bit and let mama breast feed me. Dadda went upstairs to put the pool away I was born in a birth pool, so was my big brother Alex but Alex is not the oldest Dee is. She was born in hospital and guess what! when Dadda came down Dee came too I never knew though I was busy sucking.

Jayn – waterbirth mother and founder of Splashdown, UK
When I became pregnant in May 1988 with my first baby, Nathan, I knew extremely little about birth but knew that I wanted to do the safest thing for my baby and myself, as well as the most comfortable, especially as I was going to be nearly 35 at the time of birth which was on 20 January, 1989. I knew pregnancy was not an illness so when my midwife friend suggested that home birth was probably safer than going into hospital, especially if I did not want to take medical pain relief, I opted for this as long as there were no complications.

Whilst I was pregnant, I saw a documentary on BBC TV in August 1988 about a GP in Cornwall called Dr Roger Lichy, who used to carry a portable waterbirth pool on the roof of his car and delivered babies at home. This seemed a wonderfully natural idea to me with the baby being born into water, the only physical environment it had known. The pool seemed to ease the mother's discomfort and the experience seemed very positive for the whole family. Soon after, I also saw a full page article in the *Independent* newspaper of a baby called Sam who was born at home in a waterbirth pool to Tess, Sheila Kitzinger's daughter. There was a lovely photograph of baby Sam looking straight into his mum's eyes. This seemed the perfect birth to me and encouraged me to have a waterbirth at home.

My experience was so wonderful, with the incredible pain being totally relieved immediately on immersion into the pool, that I knew I had to encourage other mothers to choose this way of giving birth. However, there was a lack of pools available. I bought two portable waterbirth pools from the Active Birth Centre and formed a service to hire them out to mothers-to-be. I worked at Shell International at the time and when they heard about Nathan's birth a story appeared in their newspaper, 'Splashdown for Nathan'. I knew I had the perfect name for my enterprise, which I called Splashdown Water Birth Services.

In 1993 the Royal College of Obstetricians and Gynaecologists reported to the media that two babies in Bristol had drowned as a result of their mothers using waterbirth pools. Those of us involved with waterbirth *knew* this was untrue. The mothers who had given birth had only laboured in the water and not given birth in the pools at all. Indeed, photos of my Nathan were in the papers with the heading 'Death of the Water Babies'. My Nathan is now a very healthy 21-year-old! I investigated the situation and issued a press release stating my findings but the papers would not retract their story. There was only one way to bring the truth to people's attention and that was to invite everyone from around the world to London to present their information about waterbirth. The Conference was a huge success with speakers from all over the world and 1500 professionals in attendance. A lot of networking took place and research is still going on as a result of this Conference.

Although I have now moved on and now run my own Academy of Angelic Healing, I still organize Midwife Study Days regularly on waterbirth and complementary therapies. I am so very pleased to have played my part in making waterbirth more available internationally and hope its popularity continues to grow so that future generations can benefit.

Angela – midwife in a midwifery-led unit, UK

During the spring of 2007 I was asked if I would like to join the team of the new 'Midwifery-led Unit' in the hospital where I work. I had been a community midwife for a while and coming back into the consultant-based unit I found that the ideals in the hospital delivery suite, with its reliance on technology and the high incidence of Caesarean sections encountered, were not really compatible with the midwifery that I loved.

Imagine my joy when on the first day of working on the new unit I was caring for a young woman expecting her first child and keen to have a waterbirth. I must confess that I had never seen a waterbirth, let alone conducted one! However, I was under the close instruction of my supervisor of midwives who happened to be on duty with me that day.

Julie [not her real name] was very worried that she would not cope with the pain of the contractions but did not like the thought of pethidine or an epidural anaesthetic. She had heard that the new unit had opened and asked if she could have her baby there using the birthing pool. This request was supported and when she was ready she climbed into the water. The transformation was remarkable. Julie had started to panic each time a contraction came and even the entonox seemed to be losing its effect. Now, in the water, she was changed, calm and smiling. The contractions were just as strong but with the warmth and comfort of the water around her she felt much more in control of her situation. The atmosphere in the room changed from a battleground to the peace of a cathedral!

The labour progressed and Julie delivered a little boy; he floated to the surface of the water and Julie gathered him in her arms. The atmosphere in the room erupted with congratulations and laughter – happiness and relief expressed by all in the room. Apart from quiet instructions to Julie, regarding holding her baby, keeping his body under the water and head out, very little was said or done by me. I have since conducted many waterbirths on the unit. I get the same feeling of joy and wonder each time.

I will compare my experiences. On a delivery suite one is surrounded by technology: CTG machines, which are noisy; Resuscitaires, which look formidable; electronic blood pressure machines which when used make a vice-like grip on the arm of the mother; there are deadlines to keep and the delivery suite sounds like – and is – a busy place. The midwives and doctors work very hard and, quite often, because of the urgency of some of the situations, they look anxious and distressed, which is quickly picked up by the mothers and they begin to worry, which all too often leads to adverse outcomes with the labours.

On the other hand, in the Midwifery-led Unit the atmosphere is one of calm and gentleness. The only machine likely to be used is a sonic aid and even that is sometimes ignored in preference to the Pinard's trumpet! Quiet encouragement and one-to-one care is the norm and it is not unusual to see the midwife in the room chatting and drinking tea with the family who are supporting the mother.

Amy and Adam – waterbirth parents and pool company owners, UK

After disappointment in 2001 when the birthing pool in Birmingham Women's Hospital was not available for the birth of our first child, in 2003 I hired a traditional birthing pool for the birth of our second child and had a wonderful birth at our home. This experience highlighted a need in the market for affordable, easy-to-access birthing pools: pools were not widely available and were quite expensive to hire. The Good Birth Company was born – hanging its hat on value pricing and great customer service. Six months later I noticed a trend in the United States where some websites were offering paddling pools for waterbirths for a fraction of the cost of a hired pool. As an experiment, my husband and I imported 50 of these pools to test the market for budget birthing pools. The results were astounding; these pools sold almost immediately without any impact on the hired pool market! After several months of selling paddling pools, which though affordable had obvious limitations in that they were not designed for indoor use or for childbirth, we ran focus groups with midwives and mothers who had used water for labour. Our goal was to capture the best of both worlds – a purposeful and robust design of an inflatable pool for labour childbirth while maintaining the ease and affordability inflatable pools can allow. The result was Birth Pool in a Box in its current design, with three stacked independently inflated chambers, specially placed handles and a liner system which allows for fast clean-up as well as safe and hygienic use of water for birth. Our Professional Pool allows for multiple use either within the community or on the maternity unit. Some areas of the UK are now experiencing increased home birth rates as pools are being offered by NHS Trusts as part of their home birth service.

Kate – mother and doula, UK

Birth of Belinda Amy: When I got in the water, the relief was instant. The bath was quite full but I wasn't submerged – I was in my favourite all-fours position – so Marcus got a large measuring jug from the kitchen. When my next contraction began, he started scooping the water up and pouring it over my shoulders, letting it run gently down my back. As it did so, it trickled around my sides and around my bump. It felt as though I was being wrapped in the softest, warmest gentlest blanket and softly caressed. Safe. Wonderful! So wonderful in fact that far from fearing the next contraction, I was positively welcoming them. I couldn't believe that the discomfort that I had been feeling out of the water was so much easier to bear. I couldn't put it into words, I just kept saying: 'I don't believe it! The pain's gone! It's gone! I can't believe it!' It baffled me so much how a simple thing like a bath that's available to anyone could have such a dramatic effect.

The water went cold, I got out, Marcus ran another bath, I got in. In all I think I had three or four baths; each time I got in I had the same sensations when the water was poured over me – like a super security blanket!

Our cue to leave for the hospital came when my body rejected the food I'd managed to eat in a fairly dramatic way! I was slightly panicked by not being able to breathe, vomit and contract at the same time. We made our way to the hospital, arriving at about 3.00pm.

By 5.00 p.m. I was taken from the ward to the delivery ward. I insisted on being taken to the room with a pool in but was not allowed to use it as my waters had gone and were heavily bloodstained. Twenty minutes later our daughter was born naturally on the bed. Healthy and safe. The placenta arrived less than 5 minutes after in a managed third stage with the membranes slightly torn but complete.

A midwife commented to me after a while that the birth had been swift and trouble free and I might like to stay at home next time. So I did!! ...

Birth of Alexander Peter: At 11.30 my husband Marcus was home, filling the pool, and a community midwife was on her way. My contractions were about 1 in 5 and quite easy to handle with a bit of breathing and I was bustling about getting bits and pieces ready for my home waterbirth. At about 1.00 a.m. I was in the pool on all fours, using the side for support. The contractions were not difficult for me to breathe through and I felt happy and secure with Marcus and my midwife, who kept herself in the background. My conversation that had been quite chatty at first, became less and less as I settled into the rhythm of the labour and the contractions became more and more intense. The room was really quiet and I became quite lost in myself.

I really felt the buoyancy of the water and the space to move around that I'd not experienced from my previous labour in my bath and it made a difference. As the contractions intensified I was really able to broaden the reach of my knees and lower my bottom further towards the bottom of the pool, really stretching my abdomen as I felt I needed to do. I swayed my hips from side to side, rising up on my ankles and floating from one side of the pool to the other when the contractions stepped up a notch.

Thankfully I have a sense of humour! I really noticed the difference gravity made to my ability to cope out of the pool, when I went out to the bathroom. I felt so heavy I could hardly coordinate my legs for walking. How wonderful to once again surround myself in the warmth, comfort and privacy of the pool where I could transform from a clumsy fat whale to a sleek and nimble fish!

I was so relieved to once again feel the irresistible urge to push and my baby was born into the water with just a few powerful thrusts. It was 3.17 a.m. My midwife brought him to the surface and with a few poolside acrobatics (to untangle him from his long cord) I was able to hold him in my arms. There he stayed with us cooing and loving him for as long as I wanted. Then, with the cord cut, I was able to stay in the water and wait for the placenta which arrived in its own good time, into the pool at about 4.00 a.m.

This experience transformed me and empowered me in a way I could not and still cannot express. My attendants were quiet and calm and served only to empower me further. I realized for the first time, my power and strength to bring life into the world and I want to celebrate it! I felt I'd unearthed a long-kept secret. Every woman should know what she is capable of!

Birth of Eleanor Grace: Overdue again. All day I spent listening intently to my body! I was experiencing the occasional contraction that would see me having to breathe through it but then nothing for ages. My midwife said she'd visit me that evening to see I was OK and I felt a bit of a fraud – this labour was going nowhere! She told me to go to bed and chill out. Feeling disappointed and dejected, I took myself off to bed. At least make the most of a good night's sleep, I told myself.

I was restless. I couldn't get comfy. Every so often I was brought out of my slumber to reposition myself and huff and puff. I was still asleep really and felt cross that my sleep was being disturbed. Then I came round a bit more to find I had got myself into an all-fours position propped up with pillows – and I was *starving*! But I was contracting – regularly! I dared not believe it. 'I'll go downstairs and have a banana,' I told myself, and managed to eat whilst on all fours gripping the side of my empty birth pool! This had to be it! I crawled upstairs to get Marcus. It was 12.30 a.m. The midwife arrived about an hour later and Marcus was filling the pool. There was a real sense of urgency about this labour; I wanted desperately to get into the pool but had to wait for it to fill. I used my birth ball to lean on and soon found myself heading for the toilet whilst simultaneously reaching for the sick bucket! Blimey! Come on Marcus! I need that pool!

By 2.10 a.m. both my midwife and Marcus were busily pouring buckets of cold water into the pool as it had run too hot, but thankfully 5 minutes later I was immersing myself in the beautiful warmth and security of the water. Not long after that my contractions felt different, slightly pushy but it wasn't time yet in my own mind. The second midwife wasn't there it was too soon to be pushing! I managed to hold off but of course my midwife had noticed. As soon as the doorbell went, signalling the arrival of the second midwife, there was no stopping me! No time for gas, just get on with it! I desperately wanted the atmosphere to settle but my body was waiting for no one and within 3 minutes of the midwife entering the room my wonderful daughter was born! How amazing to see her for that split second immersed under the water, to plunge my arms in and lift her to my breast. She latched on and was sucking within minutes (and hasn't stopped yet, 2 years on!). It was 2.37 a.m. The cord was cut at 3.20 a.m. and I got out to deliver the placenta which arrived at 3.43. At 4 o'clock my 6-year-old daughter came down to say hello to her new baby sister. A wonderful, magical moment she will cherish, as I will, forever.

Orly – Midwife, Aquamidwifery, M.A. (in Buddhism and Eastern cultures), Israel

I was inspired and touched deeply by Cornelia Ennings' presentation 'Home Midwife and Aquamidwifery', so for the last 4 years I have been on a quest for waterbirth to be moved into Israeli labour rooms.

The task is almost fulfilled – gentle birth is moving into the Israeli system. The health ministry has approved waterbirth as a legitimate choice for women who choose to birth in a labour room under the security dome of professional staff. The doctors and midwives in the hospital where I work were inspired with the idea of waterbirth and soon our labour room will be the first one to practise it. For my midwife qualification I initiated and produced two waterbirth workshops over the last 3 years – the first one with Cornelia Enning (and also with members representing ISPPM organization promoting the dynamics and effects on unborn children in the womb). For the second workshop, as part of the education programme of the Israeli midwife association, I invited Barbara Harper and Dianne Garland for an exhilarating 2 full days of enhancing midwives from all over Israel to trust in the concept of gentle birth as an integral part of our work as hospital midwives. Moreover, I have become an Aquababy instructor and for the last 2 ½ years have worked with pregnant women in Aquayoga as a preparation for birth (breathing and wet asana), deepening the mother–unborn child connection and wellbeing. My vision is for women to find qualities of water in themselves, in their consciousness, so that pregnancy and birth will become less violent and without interventions, reflecting a peaceful and loving being for our future generation.

Madonna – return-to-practice midwife, UK

I cannot remember exactly when I first heard about waterbirths, but I clearly remember what my reaction was. I thought 'What rubbish'. This must have been in the early to mid-80s. Now here I am in 2008 promoting it.

I had been taught that the compression of the chest wall through the birthing process was an aid to respiration. Surely we were not expecting the baby to inhale fluid! After my initial reaction I gave it some thought. I knew that the baby would never knowingly be put at risk, so I was curious to find out how it worked from the physiological point of view. There was not a lot of literature around at the time. What little there was seemed to originate from Michel Odent and his practice in France.

I continued practising traditionally over the years but slowly researched waterbirths to try and enhance my understanding of the subject. This research led me to Maidstone Hospital, UK, where Dianne [Garland] practised at the time. The visit gave me answers to questions I had, and I was convinced that waterbirths were the way forward. A break in my career meant that I did not practise for 10 years. I returned 4 years ago, to find that the uptake of waterbirths was on the increase, which was quite pleasing.

I am fortunate to work on a midwife-led unit that has two birthing pools. Many women have waterbirths, although many of these women only intended to labour in water, but they found the experience so relaxing that they have decided to deliver in water. A phrase I hear often enough when a woman is in the pool is 'that feels better'.

The babies are born quite serene and placid. Most of them establish their breathing without crying, and they are content to lie in their mothers' arms and gaze.

Tonya – mother, USA

My waterbirth experience with my second child, Connor, was totally different from my first birth. For 2 weeks I had been experiencing contractions every 5 minutes for hours and I was exhausted. Unfortunately, they weren't the real thing. The morning of the 13th I called Rachel because I had been up for over 13 hours with contractions. She checked me and told me that my membranes were starting to pull away, the baby was in the right position and I was at 3 cm. Around 1.30 a.m. I woke up and realized that this was probably it. The contractions were strong and I was doubled over. Because of all of the false labour I had been experiencing I waited for a long while before waking anyone up. By 4 a.m. we agreed to meet at the birth centre. After I got off the phone with Rachel, my water broke. I was still on my knees rocking back and forth against the recliner and had a pillow in my arms, face buried in it. I was moaning through the contractions. After my water broke, there was a time of relief and this allowed me to get in the car. We were about 5 minutes away from the birth centre. As soon as we got there, my contractions intensified greatly. Rachel let us in the birth centre, got the IV going (this was an antibiotic for Group B Strep) and I laboured on the birthing ball ... contractions got very close very fast. I was very scared. My sister and sisters-in-law had their hands against the small of my back while I rocked back and forth on the birthing ball.

Rachel had the water running for the tub. When it was full enough my sister and Rachel helped me. I could barely walk and was doubled over with contractions. Rachel and Tami helped me get into the tub and wow, what a difference! I felt immediate relief from the pain. The only thing I really had to deal with in the water was the strong, almost overwhelming urge to push.

During labour I zoned everyone out, except for Rachel and her soft words of encouragement. I really progressed quite quickly. I was about 5 cm when I got into the water and a few minutes later when Rachel checked me I was at 8 cm. Then I really started to feel that I couldn't handle it anymore, I needed drugs, and that time I was ready to push. Rachel encouraged me to hang on and start pushing and she also let me know that it was too late to get medication and too late to get to the hospital. Connor was ready to be born. I believe that it was just 25 minutes after I got into the water that I was ready to really push and after just 15 minutes of gentle pushing Connor was born. I only tore a little bit outwardly and he was quite a bit larger than Kaitlyn had been. He was quiet and so alert. He was looking around and started to blink at me immediately, it was precious.

I felt great, it didn't feel as though I had just delivered an 8 lb 5.5 oz boy and honestly, I didn't feel as bad as I had after giving birth to my 7 lb 2 oz baby. Yes, I was a little bit sore, but after a few hours I felt really wonderful, almost as if I hadn't given birth. It was just a marvellous experience and one I would redo if I could. I can't speak highly enough about the need for positive encouragement and reinforcement for natural birth and the empowerment it really brings a woman. I will always be an advocate for midwives, natural birth and birth centres.

Patrick – first waterbirth father, USA, and author

Preparation for my second child's waterbirth was wide ranging. My wife and I had counselling, individually and together, as we wanted to resolve any concerns or fears we had about birth in general and the use of water. This was in 1980 and this was the first waterbirth in the USA, so no books or Google search were available. We had friends to help, doctors and midwives to interview and only one midwife wanted to be involved – that's who we employed!

I hired a portable, fibreglass jacuzzi and had 300 gallons of distilled water delivered. I transformed our garage into a beautiful waterbirth room and built a wooden framed bed next to the tub. I hung pictures on the walls, curtains and oriental rugs to make it cosy.

Katheryn's labour began suddenly and progressed quickly. She was feeling overwhelmed by the intensity of her contractions, we were enjoying the wondrous and almost mystical atmosphere we had created to welcome our child. As we immersed ourselves in the water we were enveloped by its warmth. Katheryn was relieved by the comfort and freedom of movement the water afforded her. The support team arrived at various times and quietly assumed their roles. After only a 90-minute labour Katheryn birthed Jeremy into my willing hands. Jeremy was momentarily suspended in his expanded watery world, peacefully integrating his experience. I felt privileged, humble and proud all in an instant. The three of us embraced.

We had a sense that the inner preparation we had done was central to our experience. We were unencumbered and available for every aspect of the birth of our child. We felt like we had participated in a miracle.

Sylph – mother, Canada

Our daughter, Ever Light Bloom, was born on July 22, 2008, at 4.34 p.m. in Ajax, Ontario, Canada, in the home of a very kind doula, who offered us this safe space in which to birth our baby unassisted by any professional birth attendants. She weighed 6 lb 3oz., was 19.5 inches in length, and her head measured 33 cm.

I awoke in the night several times in the wee hours of July 21, with slightly crampy contractions, but I knew instinctively that it would be quite a while still, so I went back to sleep in order to be well rested for the main event.

Later I decided then that it was time to go back inside, so that I would be near the birthing pool when I needed to get in. I settled myself on the little inflated seat at one end of the pool, and continued having contractions 3–5 minutes apart, and maintaining my composure with deep breathing and peppermint oil. Rob was wonderful, sticking close to me, and making himself available for anything I needed. He held me and spoke softly, and rocked with me through the rushes as they became stronger. At one point, maybe about 15 minutes before Ever crowned, I felt my water break, which I quietly announced. Rob commented that it was a fitting time for it to happen, since the way I was rocking in the water had just made him think of the ocean! At that point, the pain increased dramatically, and instead of just breathing through the final three contractions, I had to yell, in order to vent some of the energy that was now flowing so violently through my body! I also found that I was no longer content with merely rocking back and forth, as I had been before, but had begun bouncing up and down, holding onto the pool's sturdy handles, and making big waves in the pool. Toward the end of each of these rushes, my screams turned into long, reso-nant hums, sounding something like 'Ohhhhmmmm', and Rob joined his voice with mine, to sing our little one into the world.

With the second-to-last rush, I pushed purposefully, in unison with the contraction of my womb, and felt the baby's head come out very fast. There was just a few seconds of wondering if I could withstand the pressure, or if something was going to rupture within me, and then her head was there, with its crown facing Rob, who positioned his hands in readiness to catch her. Then with the next rush, I pushed again, with just about as much pain as when she had crowned, and she flew like a tiny torpedo, out into the water, and into her father's eager hands!

Ever's face broke the surface of the water, and her eyes blinked tenta-tively as I brought her up and leaned her against my belly, where I held her securely until the cord stopped pulsing, and she began to sputter and cough, and fuss very mildly, as her lungs began their life's work. I immedi-ately felt contractions begin, and thought the placenta would come right away, but it was over an hour and a half before I delivered it, still sitting in the pool, to which we had to add more warm water, in order to keep Ever from getting chilly. Ever nursed on my breast to see if more nipple stimula-tion would move the placenta along. Some of my helpers seemed anxious about the late arrival of the afterbirth, but I was insistent that I would remain in the water until it came out on its own, and that everything would be fine.

We left the placenta attached to Ever for 2 days, when we finally cut it at about 2 inches from her umbilicus, because the cord had become so stiff and kinked that we feared she would hook it with her feet and pull it off roughly. The last of the cord stump fell off in the bath a week after her birth.

Ever is a joy to us all, and her birth a reminder of the power and simplicity of this lovely life we are living.

Emily – student midwife, UK

As a student midwife, a waterbirth is almost like the Holy Grail of experience. You know that it exists; you can spend hours talking about it with colleagues, researching the topic in books and journals and now thanks to the internet, have relatively easy access to videos depicting waterbirth online. All you have to do is be in the right place at the right time in the right hospital with the right midwife. I was fortunate enough to cross all the boxes in the latter part of my first year of training and witness a waterbirth facilitated by Dianne Garland.

I feel that I can truly say that no matter how many books or articles you have read, or videos you have seen, the awe-inspiring reality of a waterbirth is overwhelming. Even though I had spent the time researching and discussing waterbirth, being a first-year student who had to that point only experienced high-risk labour and delivery, I had never fully considered the role of the midwife in a low-risk situation not on dry land!

My particular experience involved a multiparous woman with two previous vaginal deliveries who felt that she would benefit from the relaxing, supportive qualities of the water. When she got in the pool, the look on her face could only be described as that of pure bliss. Within the quiet of the room she was calm, soothed and was able to become fully in tune with her own body and labour.

I remember whispering to Dianne, 'What do we do now?' to which she smiled and replied, 'We watch.' For me, this concept of simply observing a labour from the sidelines was completely new but I was amazed at how much I learnt by simple observation. There was no need for a vaginal examination to assess progress, or any other monitoring, as every sign of the mother's progression was clearly visible as she laboured almost in silence and without the need for any further pain relief. The fetal heart was easily auscultated using a waterproof sonic aid, with minimal disruption to the woman, and the temperature of the pool was altered simply as required.

Though I had been left completely astonished by how much of a difference the water made as an analgesic and as support, nothing could quite prepare me for the sight of a woman delivering her own baby, in her own time, as her urges dictated. There was no need for us to support the perineum and the woman controlled the birth of the head herself. It also appeared that the stretching, burning sensation on the perineum that most women describe as the head is delivering was lessened by the water. The head restituted, the shoulders delivered without difficulty and the mother brought the baby to the surface of the water. It cried immediately and was later given Apgars of 10/1 and 10/5. The woman's sense of self-esteem and achievement was incredible, and contagious too, as I felt so happy for her and could not even begin to imagine how good she must have felt doing it on her own, being empowered by the relaxing state initiated by being in the pool.

A year on and I have not yet witnessed anything like the birth I saw that day and I think it is entirely owing to the qualities and benefits the water lent to the labour and delivery. Even though I have only ever been witness to one birth in water during my short time in the midwifery world, when speaking to a woman antenatally, I can quite often be heard to ask: 'Have you considered using water for labour and birth?'

Emma – mother, UK

Deep in the heart of Denvilles, Hampshire: About 10.30 p.m. on Sunday 24 February Emma felt a change in the expansions around her abdomen, of the type that said 'we are not going to stop until baby is born'. She didn't want to wake up Steve, but excitement took over and she urgently whispered 'Steve, Steve! I think you might want to start filling the pool up.' For the records, Steve had been filling and emptying the pool for about a week by now, to avoid using hideous chemicals to keep the still water fresh and clean.

On the borders of North Bersted: Caroline was interrupted by the welcome ring of the telephone. A far-off voice said: 'I think this is definitely labour, well, I woke Steve up just after 11 to fill the pool and I feel bad calling you just after midnight.' I asked if Emma wanted me to come over and she vaguely suggested that I 'could come over in an hour or two' … a big surge took Emma's voice away and Steve took over the phone call and we agreed I should be over within an hour.

The house was calm and still. Emma's son Ben was fast asleep.

Emma asked if the pool was ready. There was urgency in her voice which said that it was time to sink into water. Upstairs she walked, and sat on the loo. She wanted to pee, before getting into the pool, but couldn't. So Caroline told her it was safe to pee in the pool. Steve helped Emma climb over the high sides of the pool and she sank with relief into the warmth of the water. Steve came in and hugged and kissed Emma. The atmosphere was positive and gentle, just right for a baby to be born into. Steve asked Emma if he should call the midwife, but Emma did not feel it was time.

Emma changed positions, and then sat on her bottom. She found this very comfortable, and then remembered labouring in the same position with Ben. Not wanting to repeat her first labour, which ended with a ventouse extraction, she moved, changing position from squats to knees to hanging off the side of the pool. It was hurting Emma, and Caroline said 'It hurts now, then it will hurt more and then it will be so much easier.' Caroline suggested that Emma lower the tone of her voice to an 'uhhhhhhhhh'. Then Emma could feel the head, and some membrane too, that floated around in the water. Emma felt and thought 'that's not the head, that's grungy!' Then she realized what she was feeling, and her face broke into an ecstatic ray of triumphant joy. Emma cried out in joy, 'I'm doing it. I'm doing it!!' Then she spoke words of welcoming encouragement to her baby.

Emma did not want to move in case she hurt her baby and her body took a short break before building up for another surge. She slipped to one side, was pulled back by Caroline and then held onto Caroline's neck as another surge pushed out the shoulders, followed by the body, arms and legs. It was 3.45 a.m. on Monday 25 February 2008. Baby floated at the bottom of the pool, with arms and legs apart like a starfish. Emma instinctively scooped her baby up into her arms to greet her, quietly calm.

At the same time, Steve felt a drop of water on his lip. With such a dry sky, and Orion so clearly in sight, he knew that his baby had been born, so he and Ben headed back home. Father and son arrived within minutes, to meet daughter and sister, and the family was fully together. Within minutes, their midwife, Eleanor, arrived. Emma got out of the pool when the cord stopped pulsating, and Caroline and Ben wove a tie for baby's umbilical cord, which Steve then cut. Hannah had latched on beautifully and was happily breast feeding.

After Eleanor left, Emma was tucked up in bed with Hannah, ready to start their new lives together.

Lyndsey – clinical lead midwife, UK

Introducing waterbirth within a busy consultant-led unit has been challenging at times but also a real pleasure. We have developed from a unit with only a few midwives with waterbirth experience to one where there are very few who have not been involved in supporting a woman using water for labour and birth.

A lot of time, energy and commitment have resulted in a hugely successful waterbirth service and we now boast large numbers of highly skilled and experienced midwives. On the delivery suite we try to offer the use of the birthing pool before drugs and encourage all women who fit the entry criteria to use water for managing labour pain.

One of the greatest joys of being involved with this project has been listening to the birth stories of the couples who come to our antenatal education sessions: we offer the opportunity for expectant couples to come along and learn about the benefits of using water for labour and birth, watch a DVD on waterbirth and listen and talk to other couples. This has been an important part of women feeling confident in their ability to give birth the way they choose.

Supporting women using the pool has been a privilege. They have been inspiring and we have learnt a tremendous amount about physiological birth; as a result I believe our midwives feel more confident encouraging normal birth and knowing how they can facilitate a quiet, peaceful, undisturbed beautiful birth.

Linda – VBAC mother, UK

Most midwives and every obstetrician caring for me would have advised me to have an elective Caesarean section as the following shows that I am classified as a very 'high risk' mother:

FPH – 1986 – Rebecca – EMLSCS – PIH/PET – 6 lb 8 oz
FPH – 1988 – Richard – EMLSCS – Fetal distress (diagnosed as CPD) – 6 lb 8 oz
RLH – 1990 – Mathew – SVD* – 7 lb 12 oz – POP
SPH – 1993 – Suzannah – EMLSCS – Cord prolapse – 9 lb 2 oz
FPH – 2000 – Eloise – SVD – 9 lb 9 oz

... however, the team of midwives gave me superb care, which can be found in isolated pockets around the UK.

A midwife arrived and on examination I was only partially effaced and 2–3 cm dilated – this meant that it could have been hours before anything happened! It was going to be a long, latent labour.

The contractions continued all day at the same rate and for the same duration; as a distraction I decided to cut the grass in my back garden.

The next morning the contractions returned to their normal pattern of once every 5 minutes and lasting 45–50 seconds. I changed the battery in the TENS machine and continued to 'waddle' around tidying up and cleaning the house between contractions. At midday I found that I could not cope with just my TENS machine so I started to use the entonox and it greatly helped me to cope with the worst contractions; up to this point my labour had been four good, strong contractions followed by three to four mild ones, and they were still only 4–5 minutes apart!

I did say that should she [the midwife] find that I had not progressed, then I wanted to go to the hospital for artificial rupture of my membranes as I had had enough of these contractions that were not actually doing anything! When my midwife examined me several hours later I was 8 cm dilated. There was no way she was leaving me to go and get more entonox; instead she grabbed her phone and called for the supervisor of midwives and her colleague just in case the supervisor did not make it to the house in time.

Barry started to top up the pool with hot water. I had two contractions while standing up, but with the third one, my legs gave way as they felt like they were made of jelly; by now I was kneeling on the floor holding onto the entonox mask and the boost button on my TENS machine. Once the other midwife arrived at 2.40 p.m., my TENS machine was taken off my back and I got in the warm water – it was lovely!

I was still using the entonox and I was aware that the supervisor of midwives arrived at 3.00 p.m.; I found that leaning forward onto the side of the pool was a very comfortable position. The midwives were behind me. They were using a small torch and Barry's shaving mirror to see how I was progressing. At 3.10 I felt my membranes rupture spontaneously with a very distinctive 'popping' sensation. I only remember having to push three or four times before I felt a head emerge; I moved so I was leaning slightly more backwards and when I looked down I could see a head and shoulder between my legs. The midwife slipped the cord over the head and the rest of the baby's body was delivered. My baby was put onto my chest and I sat back to cuddle the baby and it was then that I was told I had a son.

The midwife was concerned that the water was a little cold for the baby, and as soon as his cord had stopped pulsating it was clamped and cut by the midwife. James was already wrapped in a towel and Barry was holding him, whilst I was left in the water until the placenta was delivered – this occurred naturally after only 10 minutes.

I did it! I've achieved my ultimate dream, a waterbirth at home.

These other areas of learning that follow can be transferred to and from most areas of clinical practice. I have included them to highlight ways of developing your own unique learning guide, which can grow as your experiences with waterbirth expand.

Literature Review

Literature reviews can be used as a basis for initial or ongoing investigation. Many organizations have their own databases, including MIDIRS, Royal College of Midwives and my own website. They act as a good starting point to find information on research, clinical practice and anecdotal stories from practitioners and parents.

Newsletters

I have seen these used in a very positive way, identifying colleagues who have undertaken their first waterbirth. Units have also identified when they have supported mother at home or following a VBAC. They are a good way of keeping practitioners up to date with any ongoing audits, and 'hot gossip' stories from home and abroad – in fact, any item of interest on the waterbirth front.

Skills Drills

With the introduction of water pools the inevitable occurred: midwives became concerned about emergency evacuation from the pool. When I teach about 'What ifs …?' (see Chapters 6 and 7) I always advise midwives about what to consider in these situations. However, nothing is black and white in our work, so they are only ever suggestions. One difference with emergency evacuation is that it needs to be well practised and a policy needs to be designed in conjunction with staff responsible for moving and handling.

My skills drills include:

- getting the pool and room ready
- ensuring appropriate equipment to assist the midwife's positions around the pool
- undertaking procedures – fetal heart auscultation, vaginal examinations and so on
- dealing with problems such as nuchal cord or shoulder dystocia
- knowing how to undertake emergency evacuation.

So, whilst the last issue always raises the greatest concern, there are many more which will assist midwives with waterbirth practice.

Competencies

These have been designed in both the USA and UK to provide more evidence for practitioners to identify their own competency in waterbirths. In the UK I identify multi-professional working, skills in third stage physiology, and understanding the newborn's first breath as some of the competencies.

Internet Alerts

One of the most useful ways of maintaining contact with the world of waterbirths is to set up an internet alert. Most days I receive alerts from my search engine that range from birth stories, to medical reviews, to problems with waterbirths. The search engine ensures that any waterbirth mention worldwide is easy to access and possibly investigate; and of course it is an opportunity to reflect on any practice issues.

Here are some examples gathered over the past few years:

- birth stories – new waterbirth centres worldwide; Portugal's first waterbirth
- medical reviews
- issues with waterbirths – hypoplastic left heart syndrome (undiagnosed)
- celebrity waterbirths.

Videos/DVDs

The beauty of a video or DVD is not just in its value for teaching, but also in the way that you can re-use and review the pictures. I have highlighted in the final chapter some of the DVDs that are on the market, and which you may find of use.

Reflective Practice

Campbell (2004) gives an example of reflective critical incident analysis following a waterbirth. She identifies a simple model known to many midwives as the Gibb reflective cycle. The article explores practical issues (such as water depth) empowering mothers, and midwives' own thoughts on supporting a mother who wishes to labour/deliver in water.

Ockenden (2001) wrote about using water for labour and delivery and highlighted several issues (research versus audit, strict criteria for use) but also gave midwives a list of suggestions to assist in using water:

- promote the benefits to women
- attend training sessions
- promote the benefits to colleagues.

Her final statement reflects well my own attitude to water: 'The under-use of pools is a multiple misfortune. It is a waste of resources, a lost opportunity for many women to improve their experience of giving birth, and also for many midwives to improve their job satisfaction.'

With reflection we can identify areas of good and not such good practice, self-awareness, training issues, actual clinical scenarios and any further investigation which will assist in utilizing water in our practice. When I was a supervisor of midwives (providing a supportive role to midwives and mothers), I encouraged midwives to reflect on their day's activities.

We might want to ask ourselves questions such as these:

- 'Why did I not offer water to a particular mother?'
- 'Did I feel supported by my colleagues when I wanted to offer physiological third stage?'
- 'Was my intuition correct in asking the mother to leave the water in second stage?'

The last question is really invaluable as it is often midwifery intuition which is undervalued by our own colleagues. You cannot teach intuition; it comes with experience and reflection, and acts as a credible rationale for areas of care where a definitive answer is not always available. With intuition we use all our senses and skills; we react when it is difficult to use a black-and-white approach to actions we undertake.

Professional Visits

Many units around the world are very happy for colleagues to visit. I have been fortunate that as a lecturer I have been able to visit birth facilities whilst teaching. I have also encouraged students that I work with to use their elective period during training to seek out different birth environments. Many units welcome visitors either for just a day or for a week, and during this time I have a professional visit pro forma I complete and keep on file (see Figure 10.1 for an example).

PROFESSIONAL VISIT

Contact name: ....
Unit/Address: ....
....
....
....

Client group: ....
Cost of service: ....
   Do parents have to hire pool/pay for liners? ....
   What type of pool is available to mothers? ....
   Is there a list of hire companies? ....
Primip vs. multip ratio: ....
What antenatal preparation is available?
General or specific classes .... Yoga .... Aquanatal ....
Are guidelines for practice available?
   Are these multi-professional? ....
   Do they include criteria for exclusion? ....
   Is TOS allowed to labour/deliver? ....
   Is risk assessment undertaken? ....
Caregivers:
   Midwife ....
   Doctor ....
   Doula ....
Additives to water: ....
   Use of aromatherapy oils..
Water temperature at labour/delivery? ....
Monitoring/base CTG: ....
Third stage management:
   In or out of water..
   Active or physiological ....
Outcomes:
   Length of labour: ....
   Perineal trauma (episiotomy under water): ....
   Apgar scores ....
   NICU admissions..
   PPH ....
Emergencies/adverse outcomes (water emboli, emergency evacuation): ....
....
....
Comments: ....
....
....
....

Figure 10.1 Professional visit pro forma

Research Relevant to Practice
The importance of educational support from skilled practitioners was highlighted by Nicoll et al. (2004).   This short article discusses how a small maternity unit in Montrose, Scotland, made positive moves to improve a 21 per cent delivery rate of local mothers. To ensure the viability of this unit, the midwives positively and proactively encouraged low-risk mothers to use water within the unit. They invited other local midwives who had waterbirth experience to run a workshop where the pros and cons of using water were discussed. This was multi-professional education supported by a professional development midwife from Tayside and representatives from AIMS (Association for Improvement in Maternity Services).

Midwifery Quiz

Table 10.1 lists mothers or babies with conditions that have warranted the question 'Can I still use water for labour or birth?' Decide for yourself in each case whether the mother may use water for labour, birth or third stage. Remember that for a woman with high BMI, water may be beneficial for labour but she would need risk assessment regarding giving birth in water; for another, water might be suitable for labour and birth but not third stage, if she had had a previous third stage problem.

Table 10.1 Midwifery quiz

	Labour	Birth	Third stage
IVF conception			
Previous LSCS			
Previous neonatal death/stillbirth			
Grand multip			
Maternal age < 15 years			
Maternal age > 45 years			
Maternal weight > 15 stone			
Mother deaf/hearing impaired			
Twins			
Breech			
Gestational diabetic			
Epileptic mother			
DVT on pill			
Myomectomy			

Table 10.1 *continued*

	Labour	*Birth*	*Third stage*
Haemoglobinopathies			
Hb < 10			
Maternal antibodies			
APH at 22/40			
Pregnancy-induced hypertension			
Pre-eclampsia			
Post-mature > 42/40			
Previous long labour			
Previous precipitate delivery			
Previous third-degree tear			
Previous episiotomy			
Previous retained placenta			
Known HIV/hepatitis mother			
Vulval varicosities			
Previous history of herpes			
Symphysis pubis dysfunction			
Umbilical hernia			
Latex allergy			
Baby with tracheo-oesophageal fistula			
Baby with kidney disease			
Perforated fundus at ToP			
Soft systolic murmur			
Congenital dislocation of hips			
Active measles			
Low thyroid levels			
Fragmin for DVT antenatally			
Previous major analgesia anaphylaxis			
Arachnoid cysts in fetal cranium			
Myalgic encephalomyletis			
Baby with ventriculomegaly			
Mother with thalassaemia trait			
IUD at 38/40			
Titanium rods at thoraic level			
Polyhydramnios			
Baby with cleft lip and palate			
Tetrology of Fallot (cardiac wall defect)			
Marfan's syndrome (stature overgrowth)			
Active genital herpes			
Fetal heart rate –? congenital arrhythmia			
'Slipped' discs – L5–S1			
Mother – congenital heart disease			
Von Willibrand's disease (clotting disorder F VIII)			
Pelvic mass – teratoma / dermoid cyst			
Brain tumour			
Classical Caesarean section scar			

	Labour	*Birth*	*Third stage*
Female circumcision			
Glaucoma			
Protein S deficiency			
Supra-ventricular tachycardia			
Latex allergy			
Baby with known trisomy 21 (Down's syndrome)			
Mother with full leg amputation			
Raynaud's syndrome			
Methadone therapy			
Endometriosis			

Questions for Discussion and Reflection

- What ongoing professional education do you believe that you may require and how are you going to achieve this?
- Look back at the case studies of experiences and reflect on the following questions:
  - Which of these women would you feel happy to offer a water labour or birth to?
  - Which would you offer a dry land or 'active' rather than water third stage to?
  - Which mothers do you feel should not be offered water at all, and why?

Use your clinical judgement and experience, review local guidelines and current dry land practice; ask your colleagues for their opinions. In some cases there is not always a definitive answer – but be ready to challenge and be challenged.

11

Help and Further Resources

Many organizations and individuals exist who are very willing to share ideas, stories and resources surrounding the use of water. I list below useful resources that cover pool hire, aquanatal classes, waterbirth equipment, DVDs and videos, and leaflets, all of which will give you a good opportunity to access wide learning. Please also visit my own website: www.midwifeexpert.com

Pool Hire

There are many units – midwife and consultant led – that have pools installed. They may be plumbed in or portable; listed below are some of the pool companies in the UK. Many of these companies have agreements with international organizations, thus expanding the availability to mothers in other countries.

In 2005 Sheila Kitzinger reminded us that in a survey in 1993 only 43 per cent of UK units offered birthing pools. Whilst that number has improved considerably, there are still many units which only offer a restricted service based on staff availability and training issues. With the resources now available, plus government direction and mothers' requests, I hope that we will soon reach a situation whereby all mothers will have the option to use water in various care settings.

The following websites are companies which offer hire or purchase of pools. The websites all have waterbirth information which may be useful to parents – especially as many are run by people who themselves have had waterbirths.

www.activebirthpools.com
www.aquabirths.co.uk
www.birthpoolinabox.co.uk
www.febromed.de

www.gentlewater.co.uk
www.waterbirth.org
www.waterbirthsolutions.com

Aquanatal Classes

These websites will give guidance on finding a local aquanatal class, and on what to expect when you attend.

www.aquanatal.be
www.aquanatal.co.uk
www.aqua-vie.com
www.birthlight.com
www.northernfitness.co.uk

General Information

These websites offer general information, and equipment or personnel who may be useful to midwives when they start supporting waterbirths. The equipment has been designed either by midwives or in close collaboration with midwives who offer waterbirths.

General

Complementary therapies: www.expectancy.co.uk
Doulas: www.doula.org.uk
General midwifery issues: www.midwiferytoday
Hypnobirthing: www.begintolive.co.uk
Independent midwives: www.independentmidwives.org.uk
VBAC: www.vbac.co.uk
Yoga: www.yogabirth.org

Equipment

Emergency evacuation net: www.silvalealtd.co.uk
Telemetry monitoring: www.cardiac-services.com
    www.philips.com/healthcare
Underwater dopplers: www.restomed.com
    www.huntleigh-diagnostics.com
Underwater mirror: www.kentmidwiferypractice.co.uk

Waterbirth learning game: Medical illustrations, Royal Wolverhampton NHS Trust, New Cross Hospital, Wolverhampton WV10 0QP

DVDs and Videos

I have highlighted some of the many waterbirth/alternative birth DVDs and videos which I use when teaching. They may challenge our views of birth or provide a valuable resource to learning, and can be used in parent education classes.

The Art of Birth: The Story of Four Gentle Births in Water by S. Caplice and T. Dusseldorp. Contact at: shea@bigpond.net.au

Birth in Water by Dr Andrew Davidson. Contact him at: adavidson@adavidson.com.au

Born in Water: A Sacred Journey. www.waterbirth.net

Birth as We Know It by Elana Tonetti-Vladimirova. www.Birthintobeing. com

Gentle Birth Choices by Barbara Harper. www.waterbirthsolutions.com

A Guide to Water Birth by Ethel Burns. Oxford Medical Illustration, John Radcliffe Hospital, Oxford, OX3 9DU

Orgasmic Birth by Debra Pascal-Bonaro. www.orgasmicbirth.com

Underwater Delivery in the 21st Century: The Aquanatal Experience in Ostend. www.aquanatal.be

The Use of Water for Labour and Birth by Marina Alzugaray (video). www.midwiferytoday.com/videos/waterlabor.asp

Leaflets

Association for Improvement in Maternity Services. *Choosing a Waterbirth*. wwwaims.org.uk

Midwives Information and Resource Service. *Do You Want a Waterbirth?* www.midirs.org

National Childbirth Trust. *Labour and Birth in Water*. www.nctpregnan-cyandbabycare.com

Concluding Comment ...

I finish with a quote from an unknown sixteenth-century midwifery text:

A midwife should possess a lady's hand
A hawk's eye
And a lion's heart.

These aspects are all essential in midwifery practice. They have been vital aspects of my own attidude to care and have assisted me as I have moved through my journey with waterbirth.

I wish you well with your own exploration of waterbirth. I have learnt so much from mothers, midwives, doctors and the huge range of colleagues whom I have met over the past 24 years of waterbirth. Use this book in the way it has been written – with love, skill and knowledge.

Appendix 1

Effects of Adrenaline and Noradrenaline on All Major Systems

	Adrenaline 80%	Noradrenaline 20%
Effects on nervous system	Wakefulness Emotionality	Anxiety

Effects on cardiovascular system	Cardiac output
	Peripheral resistance
	Increased systolic blood
	    pressure
	Increased diastolic blood
	    pressure
		Increased blood pressure
		Pallor
		Sweat
		Anxiety

Effects on respiratory system	Increased metabolic rate Energy utilization Heat production Oxygen consumption	

Adrenaline and noradrenaline are secreted from the adrenal medulla. Feedback is via nerve impulses to the hypothalamus. Increased adrenaline levels are observed with hypothermia and hypoglycaemia.

Hans Selye's general adaption system introduced a system to show the three phases of alleged effects of stress on the body. More up-to-date references include:

Greenberg, N. et al. 2002. Causes and consequences of stress. *Integrated and Complementary Biology* 42: 508–16.

Lothian, J. 2004. Do not disturb – the importance of privacy in labor. *Journal of Perinatal Education* 13(3) Summer: 4–6.

Mayes, L. C. 1994. Understanding adaptive processes in a developmental context. *Psychoanalytic Study of the Child* 49: 12–35.

Appendix 2

Hyperthermia

In studies undertaken on pregnant ewes there is some evidence that maternal hyperthermia could have a profound effect on fetal temperature and heart rate (Cefalo et al. 1978). Heat application to the uterus whilst contracting appears to cause an accelerated local metabolic rate and arteriolar dilation (Khamis et al. 1983). With this in mind, it is worth reviewing the adult mechanism of heat balance regulation and the effects of hyperthermia.

Heat Regulation

- Control is via the anterior hypothalamus, which protects against overheating and overcooling.
- Long-term heat adjustments involve the pituitary, thyroid and adrenal glands.

Hypothalmus

Anterior region: The optic chiasma and anterior commissure prevent overheating; they assist through vasodilation and sweating.

Posterior region: The corpora mammillaria protects from cold; assists through vasoconstriction and shivering.

There is an interplay between the two lobes. Maintenance of the core temperature at 37 °C is through peripheral thermoreceptors in the skin and the reflex that occurs at this level, and hyporeceptors via circulating blood (Bazett, cited Newburgh 1968).

Heat Gain

- Metabolism: increased tissue metabolism occurs with exercise to 39 °C and is affected by circulating thyroxine.
- External environment: increases the core temperature if the ambient temperature is greater.
- Hot foods and drinks cause a minimal rise in temperature.

Hormones

Hormones that can cause a rise in temperature:

- Thyroxine – little effect
- Adrenaline – in a hot environment adrenaline is secreted into the blood stream. Its function is to cause modifications to the blood supply in favour of muscle (uterus), liberation of glucose, which can be assimilated, and an increase in heat production.
- Noradrenaline
- Progesterone – little effect

Heat Loss

Eighty-five per cent of heat loss occurs through conduction and convection:

- Conduction – little loss through cooler direct surface contact. Heat conducted from within the body to the skin surface and out to any cooler surface.
- Convection – heat transfer is dependent upon physical transfer of a liquid or gas. Streams of air rise from a warm surface. Increased air circulation causes increased convection.
- Radiation – the exchange of thermal energy between objects, through a process which depends only upon the temperature and the nature of the surfaces of the radiating objects. Heat passes through the skin to other objects in its path.
- Evaporation – water evaporates from the body via the skin and lungs. If the skin is moist then there is increased evaporation. Skin-to-air exchange occurs a few millimetres from the skin surface, thus

there is not an ambient temperature; with stagnant air this energy transfer may be reduced.

- Water loss also occurs into the environment through sweating.
- Minimal loss also occurs through urine/faeces and the respiratory tract.

Appendix 3

Temperature Control Pathway for the Fetus *in Utero*

Fetal temperature is approximately 0.5 °C above the mother's. Heat accumulates in the fetal body and surrounding amniotic fluids. The differential between the mother's and baby's temperature allows this heat to pass to the mother through the umbilical circulation, fetal skin and amniotic fluid to the placenta and thus the uterine wall (Power 1989). Figure A.1 shows this in diagrammatic form.

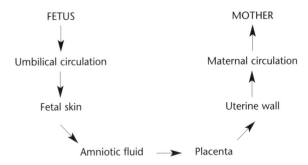

Figure A1   Diagram of fetal heat loss

Effects of Hydrotherapy and Hyperthermia

	Midwifery care	*Pathology*
Normal heat adaptation		
Conduction	Water temperature	Dehydration
Convection	Maternal temperature	Hyperthermia
Radiation	Ambient room temperature	Tachycardia
Evaporation	Free fluids	Increased metabolic rate
	Water depth	
	Time limit	

	Midwifery care	Pathology
Fetal heat adaptation		
Placenta and amniotic fluid	Heart rate auscultation	Tachycardia Hyperthermia Increased oxygen requirements/cerebral compromise
Compounded by labour hypoxia		Pathological anoxia

Further Reading

Anim–Somuah, M., R. M. D. Smyth, and C. J. Howell. 2005. Epidural versus non-epidural or no analgesia in labour. Cochrane database of systematic reviews. Issue 4 Art. No CD000331.

Balaskas, J. 2004. *The Waterbirth Book*. London: Thorsons.

Burns, E. and S. Kitzinger. 2000. *Midwifery Guidelines for Use of Water in Labour*. Oxford: OCHRAD.

Coad, J. and M. Dunstall. 2005. *Anatomy and Physiology for Midwives*. UK: Mosby.

Freedman, F. B. 2000. *Aquayoga*. USA: Lorenz Books.

Freedman, F. B. 2008. *Aqualight*. UK: Birthlight.

Government of South Australia Department of Health. 2005. *Policy – Birth in Water*.

Gradert, Y. et al. 1987. Warm tub during labour. *Acta Obstetricia et Gynecologica Scandinavica* 66: 681–3.

Harper, B. 2000. Waterbirth basics: from newborn breathing to hospital protocols. *Midwifery Today* 54: 9–15.

Harper, B. Forthcoming. *The Complete Guide to Waterbirth*.

Hess, S. 2005. Strong opinions versus science in waterbirth controversy. *Pediatrics* 116(2) August: 522–3.

Howsen, P. M. 2007. *Fathers-to-be Handbook*. UK: Creative Life Systems.

Johnson, J. and M. Odent. 1994. *We Are All Waterbabies*. London: Dragons World.

Johnston, M. 2008. Death of newborn baby – avoidable – doctor. *New Zealand Herald*, 3 July. nzherald.co.nz

Lawrence, K. 2009. Joyous birth advocate's child birth death tragedy. *Daily Telegraph* (Australia), 6 April.

Levine, B. A. 1984. Use of hydrotherapy in reduction of anxiety. *Psychological Reports* 55: 526.

Marchant, S. et al. 1996. Labour and birth in water – national variations. *BMJ* 20: 79–85.

Meyer, S. L. et al. 2010. Perceptions and practice of waterbirth: a survey of Georgia midwives. *Journal of Midwifery and Women's Health* 55(1): 55–9.

Nyuyen, S. et al. 2002. Waterbirth, a near drowning experience. *Pediatrics* 110: 411–13.

Odent, M. 1984. *Birth Reborn*. London: Fontana Collins.

Parker, P. et al. 1995. Pseudomonas otitis media and bacteremia after a waterbirth. *Pediatrics* 99(4): 653.

Perez-Botella, M. and S. Downe. 2006. Stories as evidence: why do midwives still use directed pushing? *British Journal of Midwifery* 14(10) October: 596–9.

Rawal, J. et al. 1994. Birthing tub caused infection. *Nursing Times* 90(35) 31 August.

Ridgeway, G. et al. 1996. Birthing pools and infection control. *Lancet* 347: 1051–2.

Roome, A. et al. 1996. Birthing pools and infection control. *Lancet* 348: 274–5.

Tuteur, A. 2009. What's in the water at waterbirth? 19 November 2009 www.Sciencebasedmedicine.org (accessed 13 July 2010).

Walker, J. 1994. Birth underwater: sink or swim. *British Journal of Obstetrics and Gynaecology* 101: 467–8.

References

Ahmed, M. A. and A. D. Patel. 2005. Bilateral neuropraxia of the common peroneal nerve following water birth delivery. *Injury Extra* 37(5) May: 208–10.

Alderdice, F. et al. 1995. Labour and birth in water in England and Wales. *British Journal of Midwifery* 310: 837.

Aldrich, C. D. d'Antionia, J. Spence, J. Wyatt, D. Peebles, D. Delphy and E. Reynolds. 1995. The effect of maternal pushing on foetal cerebral oxygenation and blood volume during the second stage of labour. *British Journal of Obstetrics and Gynaecology* 102: 448–53.

Alexander, J., V. Levy and S. Roch. 1993. *Midwifery Practice: A Research Approach.* London: Palgrave Macmillan.

Amos, D. 2005. Handle with care. *The Practising Midwife* 8(5) May: 15–19.

Anderson, T. 2000. Umbilical cords and underwater birth. *The Practising Midwife* 3(2): 12.

Anderson, T. 2004. Time to throw the waterbirth thermometer away? *MIDIRS* 14(3): 370–4.

Andrews, H. R. 1914. *Midwifery for Nurses.* London: Edward Arnold.

Austin, T. et al. 1997. Severe neonatal polycythaemia after 3rd stage of labour underwater. *The Lancet* 350 (15 November): 1145.

Baddeley, S. 1999. Client health aquanatal classes. ICM conference proceedings, Manila: ICM.

Bailey, A. 2009. Enoch's home waterbirth after four C-sections. *Midwifery Today* Spring: 14–15.

Balaskas, J. and Y. Gordon. 1992. *Waterbirth.* London: HarperCollins.

Banks, M. 2009. Waterbirth in New Zealand: her story and politics. *Birthspirit Midwifery Journal* 1 February: 13–19.

Baylies, W. 1757. *Practical Reflections on the Uses and Abuses of Bath Water.* London: Millar.

Beech, B. 1996. *Waterbirth Unplugged.* Manchester: BFM.

Benfield, R. D. et al. 2007. The psychophysiological effects of hydrotherapy on anxiety and pain in human labor. Poster presentation/personal correspondence. *Reproductive Sciences* 14(1) January: 147a.

Benko, A. 2009. Waterbirth: is it a real choice? *Midwifery Matters* 122 Autumn: 9–12.

Benyon, C. 1957/1990. The normal second stage: a plea for reform in its conduct. In S. Kitzinger and P. Simkin, *Episiotomy and the Second Stage of Labour* (2nd edn). Seattle: Pennypress.

Brook, D. 1976. *Nature Birth.* Harmondsworth: Penguin.

Brucker, M. C. 1984. Non-pharmacological methods of relieving pain and discomfort during pregnancy. *MCN* 19 November/December: 390–4.

Buckley, S. J. 2005. *Gentle Birth, Gentle Mothering.* Brisbane: One Moon Press.

Burke, H .1985. The shock of birth. *Nursing Mirror* 11 September: 161.

Burns, E. 2001. Waterbirth. *MIDIRS* 11(3) September, supplement 2: 510–13.

Burns, E. and K. Greenish. 1993. Waterbirth: pooling information. *Nursing Times* 89(8): 47–9.

Burns, E. and S. Kitzinger. 2000. *Midwifery Guidelines for Use of Water in Labour.* Oxford: OCHRAD.

Butler, R. and J. Fuller. 1998. Back pain following epidural anaesthesia in labour. *Canadian Journal of Anesthesia* 18 December: 724–8.

Byrom, A. and S. Downe. 2005. Second stage of labour: challenging the use of directed pushing. *Midwives* 8(4): 168–9.

Cain, M. 1992. Taking to the water. *Midwives Chronicle* June: 148–9.

Caldeyro-Barcia, R. 1979. The influences of maternal bearing down efforts during the second stage of labor on fetal wellbeing. *Birth and the Family Journal* 6(1): 17–23.

Cammu, H. et al. 1994. 'To bathe or not to bathe' during the first stage of labor. *Acta Obstetricia et Gynecologica Scandinavica* 73: 468–72.

Campbell, G. 2004. Critical incident analysis of water immersion. *British Journal of Midwifery* 12(1) January: 7–11.

Caroci da Costa, Adriana de souza and Maria Luiza Gonzalez Riesco. 2006. A comparison of 'hands off' versus 'hands on' techniques for decreasing perineal lacerations during birth. *Journal of Midwifery and Women's Health* 51(2): 106–11.

Cefelo, R. C. et al. 1978. The effects of maternal hyperthermia on maternal and fetal cardiovascular and respiratory function. *American Journal of Obstetrics and Gynecology* 131(6) 15 July: 687–94.

CEMACH. 2000–2. *Why Mothers Die.* 6th Report, ed. G. Lewis. London: CEMACH.

CEMACH. 2003–5. 7th report, ed. G. Lewis. London: CEMACH.

CEMACH. 2007. *Saving Mothers' Lives.* London: CEMACH.

Centres for Disease Control and Prevention. 2002. Prevention of perinatal Group B streptococcus disease. *Morbidity and Mortality Weekly Report* 51: 1–18.

Chalk, A. 2004. Spontaneous versus directed pushing. *British Journal of Midwifery* 12(10) October: 626–30.

Channel 4. 1994. *Brave New Babies – Learning before Birth.* London: Channel 4.

Charles, C. 1998. Foetal hyperthermia risk from warm water immersion. *British Journal of Midwifery* 6(3) March: 152.

Church, L. K. 1989. Waterbirths: one birthing centre's observations. *Journal of Nursing Midwifery* 34(4): 165.

Clift-Matthews, V. 2007. So much diversity in practice: Caesarean or waterbirth? *British Journal of Midwifery* 15(1) January: 4.

Cluett, E. and R. Bluff. 2006. *Principles and Practice of Research in Midwifery* (2nd edn). Oxford: Elsevier.

Cluett, E. R. and E. Burns. 2009. Immersion in water in labour and birth. Review, The Cochrane Collaboration. London: Wiley.

Cluett, E. R. et al. 2004. Randomised controlled trial of labouring in water compared with standard of augmentation for management of dystocia in first stage of labour. *BMJ* 10(1136) (26 January).

Coad, J. and M. Dunstall. 2005. *Anatomy and Physiology for Midwives.* Mosby.

Cochrane, A. and K. Callen. 1998. *Beyond the Blue.* London: Bloomsbury.

Cole, L. 2004. NACC water birth survey. *NACC News* December: 9.

Craig, R. 2010. Birth from the other side. *Midwifery Matters* 124 Spring: 10–12.

Cro, S. and J. Preston. 2002. Cord snapping at waterbirth delivery. *British Journal of Midwifery* 10(8) August: 494–7.

Cross, K. W. 1961. Head's paradoxical reflex. *Brain* 84 (part 4) December: 529–34.

Crozier, K. and M. Sinclair. 1999. Birth technology. *Midwives Journal* 2(95): 60–4.

Curtis, L. M. 1994. The aspiration of stomach contents into the lungs during obstetric anesthesia. *Survey of Anesthesiology* 38(3) June: 185.

da Silva, F. M. et al. 2007. A randomized controlled trial evaluating the effect of immersion bath on labour pain. *Midwifery* DOI 10.1016/j.midw.2007.04.006.

Davidson, A. 2002. Conference presentation – a conference about working together. UK.

Davies, L. 2009. Going with the flow – an alternative perspective on VBAC. *Birthspirit Midwifery Journal* Issue 1 February: 47–50.

Davis, E. 2004. *Heart and Hands*. Berkeley, CA: Celestial Arts.

Davison, J. S. et al. 2005. Gastric emptying time in late pregnancy and labour. *BJOG, An International Journal of Obstetrics and Gynaecology* 77(1): 37–41.

Dawes, G. 1968. *Foetal and Neonatal Physiology*. Chicago: Year Book Medical.

Deans, A. 1995. Temperature of pool is important. *BMJ* 311: 390–1.

Dick-Read, G. 1953 (reprinted 1984). *Childbirth without Fear*. New York: Perennial.

DoH (Department of Health). 1993. *Changing Childbirth*: Report of the Expert Maternity Group. London HMSO.

DoH (Department of Health). 2004. *National Service Framework for Children, Young People and Maternity Services*. London: DoH.

DoH (Department of Health). 2007. *Maternity Matters: Choice, Access and Continuity of Care in a Safe Service*. London: DoH.

DoH (Department of Health). 2008. *High Quality Care for All*, ed. Lord Darzi. London: DoH.

Doniec-Ulman, I. et al. 1987. Water immersion-induced endocrine alterations in women with EPH gestosis. *Clinical Nephrology* 28(2): 51–5.

Downe, S. 2009. Eating a light diet during labour. *BMJ* 338: b732.

Dunn, P. M. 1985. Management of childbirth in normal women: the third stage and fetal adaptation. In *Perinatal Medicine*, Proceedings of the IX European Congress of Perinatal medicine, Dublin, September 1984. Lancaster: MTP Press, pp. 47–54.

Easmon, C. S. 1986. The carrier state: group B streptococcus. *Journal of Antimicrobial Chemotherapy* 18: 59–65.

Eckert, K., D. Turnbull and A. MacLennan. 2001. Immersion in water in the first stage of labour: a randomised controlled trial. *Birth* 28(2): 84–92.

Edlich, R. F. et al. 1987. Bioengineering principles of hydrotherapy. *JBCR* 8(6): 581–5.

Eldering, G. and K. Selke. 1999. In *Waterbirth in the 21st Century*. Ostend, Belgium, pp. 24–9.

Enkin, M. et al. 2000. *A Guide to Effective Care in Pregnancy and Childbirth*. Oxford: Oxford University Press.

Enning, C. 2007. Aquamidwifery – a New Standard of European Care. Gentle Birth World Conference presentation. Portland, Oregon.

Ericksson, M. et al. 1997. Early or late bath during the first stage of labour: a randomized study of 200 women. *Midwifery* 13: 146–8.

Fairbairn, J. S. 1914. *A Text Book for Midwives*. Oxford: Oxford Medical Publications.

Falconer, A. D. and A. B. Powles. 1982. Plasma noradrenaline levels during labour. *Anaesthesia* 37: 416–20.

Falconer, W. 1770. *An Essay on Bath Water*. London: Robinson.

Farrar, D. 2009. How evidence based practice can provide the way forward for third stage care. *Midwives* December/January: 20.

Fehervary, P., E. Lauinger-Lörsch, H. Hof, F. Melchert, L. Bauer and W. Zieger. 2004. Waterbirth: microbiological colonization of the newborn, neonatal and maternal infection rate in comparison to conventional bed deliveries. *Archives of Gynaecology and Obstetrics* 270(1) July: 6–9.

Frye, A. 2004. *Holistic Midwifery*, Volume 11. Portland, OR: Labry Press.

Garland, D. 1994. Waterbirth: first stage immersion or non-immersion. *British Journal of Midwifery* 2(3): 113–20.

Garland, D. 2000a. *Waterbirth – An Attitude to Care*. Oxford: BFM.

Garland, D. 2000b. What is normal labour and birth? Personal correspondence. Christ Church College, Canterbury, UK.

Garland, D. 2002. Collaborative waterbirth audit – 'Supporting practice with audit'. *MIDIRS Midwifery Digest* 12(4): 508–11.

Garland, D. 2004. Is the use of water in labour an option for women following a previous LSCS? *MIDIRS Midwifery Digest* 14(1): 63–7.

Garland, D. 2006a. On the crest of a wave. Completion of a collaborative audit. *MIDIRS* 16(1): 81–5.

Garland, D. 2006b. Is waterbirth a safe and realistic option for mothers following a previous Caesarean section? *MIDIRS* 16(2): 217–20.

Garland, D. 2006c. Waterbirth – an international overview. *International Midwifery* 19(2): 24–5.

Garland, D. and K. Jones. 1994. Waterbirth, first stage immersion or non-immersion? *British Journal of Midwifery* 2(3): 113–20.

Garland, D. and K. Jones. 1997. Waterbirth – updating the evidence. *British Journal of Midwifery* 5(6) June: 368–73.

Garland, D. and K. Jones. 2000. Waterbirths – supporting practice with clinical audit. *MIDIRS* 10(3): 333–6.

Gaskin, I. M. 2002. *Spiritual Midwifery*. Summertown, TN: Book Publishing Company.

Gaskin, I. M. 2008. *Guide to Childbirth*. USA: Vermilion.

GBS Support. 2007. *GBS and Pregnancy*. West Sussex.

Geissbuhler, V. et al. 2000. Waterbirths: a comparative study. *Fetal Diagnosis and Therapy* 15: 291–300.

Geissbuehler, V., K. Eberhard and A. Lebrecht. 2002. Waterbirth: water temperature and bathing time – mother knows best. *Journal of Perinatal Medicine* 30: 371–8.

Geissbuehler, V., S. Stein and J. Eberhard. 2004. Waterbirths compared with landbirths: an observational study of nine years. *Journal of Perinatal Medicine* 32: 308–14.

Gilbert, R. E. and P. A. Tookey. 1999. Perinatal mortality and morbidity among babies delivered in water – surveillance study and postal survey. *BMJ* 319: 483–7.

Gillot de vries, F. et al. 1987. Influence of a bath during labor on the experience of maternity. *Pre- and Perinatal Psychology* 1(4) Summer: 297–302.

Ginesi, L. et al. 1998. Neuroendocrinology and birth: 1: stress. *British Journal of Midwifery* 6(10): 659–63.

Gould, D. 2004. Trust me, I am a midwife. *British Journal of Midwifery* 12(1) January: 44.

Gould, D. 2007. Waterbirth: from ordinary to extraordinary. *British Journal of Midwifery* 15(1) January: 4.

Gradert, Y. et al. 1987. Warm tub during labour. *Acta Obstetricia et Gynecologica Scandinavica* 66: 681–3.

Guise, J. M., M. S. McDonagh, P. Osterwell, P. Nygren, B. K. S. Chan and M. Helfand. 2004. Systematic review of the incidence and consequences of uterine rupture in women with previous Caesarean section. *BMJ* 329 (3 July): 19–23.

Gyte, G. 1992. The significance of blood loss at delivery. *MIDIRS* 2(1): 88–92.

Haggertay, H. 2008. Should midwives delay administration of syntometrine? *Midwives* 11(3): 16.

Halksworth, G. 1994. *Aquanatal Exercises*. Manchester: Books for Midwives.

Hall, S. M. and I. M. Holloway. 1998. Staying in control. Women's experiences of labour in water. *Midwifery* 14: 30–6.

Hamed, H. et al. 1967. Role of carotoid chemoreceptors in the initiation of effective breathing of the lamb at term. *Paediatrics* 39(3): 329–36.

Harper, B .1994. *Gentle Birth Choices*. USA.

Harper, B. 2000. Gentle Birth Conference. Portland, Oregon, 2000.

Harper, B. 2002. Taking the plunge: re-evaluating waterbirth temperature guidelines. *MIDIRS* 12(4) December: 506–7.

Harper, B. 2005. *Gentle Birth Choices*. Vermont: Healing Arts Press. See at www.waterbirth.org

Harris, T. 2001. Changing the focus for the third stage. *British Journal of Midwifery* 9(1) January: 7–12.

Hawkins, S. 1995 Water vs. conventional births: infection rates compared. *Nursing Times* 91(11): 38–40.

Health and Safety Executive. 2009. Control of substances hazardous to health (COSHH). London: HMSO.

Healthcare Commission. 2008. *Towards Better Birth*. London.

Heath, P. T. et al. 2004. Group B streptococcal disease in UK and Irish infants < 90 days of age. *Lancet* 363(9405): 292.

Higson, A. 2008. Cord clamping. *Midwives* 11(6): 14.

House of Commons Health Committee. 1992. Maternity Services. London: HMSO.

Howell, J. C. et al. 2002. Randomised study of long-term outcome after epidural versus non-epidural analgesia during labour. *BMJ* 17 August: 325–57.

Howsen, P. 2009. The science of 'father love'. www.Fatherstobe.org (accessed 13 July 2010).

Huntingford, P. 1985. *Birthright: The Parents' Choice*. London: BBC.

Inglis, B. and R. West. 1983. *The Alternative Health Guide*. London: Michael Joseph.

Johnson, P. 1996. Birth under water – to breathe or not to breathe? *British Journal of Obstetrics and Gynaecology* 103 March: 202–8.

Jowitt, M. 1993. Beta endorphin and stress in pregnancy and labour. *Midwifery Matters* 56 Spring: 3–4.

Kassim, Z., M. Sellars and A. Greenough. 2005. Underwaterbirth and neonatal respiratory distress. *BMJ* 330 (7 May): 1071–2.

Katz,V. L. et al. 1988. Fetal and uterine responses to immersion and exercise. *Obstetrics and Gynaecology* 72(2) August: 225–30.

Katz, V. L., R. M. Ryder, R. C. Cefalo, S. C. Carmichael and B. A. Goolsby. 1990. A comparision of bed rest and immersion for treating the edema of pregnancy. *Obstetrics and Gynecology* 75(2): February: 147–51.

Keirse, M. J. N. C. 2005. Challenging water birth – how wet can it get? *Birth* 32(4) December: 318–22.

Khamis, Y. et al. 1983. Effect of heat on uterine contractions. *International Journal of Gynaecology and Obstetrics* 21: 491–3.

Kiran, T. S. U. and N. S. Jayawickrama. 2002. Who is responsible for the rising Caesarean section rate? *Journal of Obstetrics and Gynaecology* 22(4): 363–5.

Kirkham, M. 2009. Home Birth conference. Chichester, UK.

Kitzinger, S. 2000. Letter from Europe – the waterbirth debate up to date. *Birth* 27(3): 214–16.

Kitzinger, S. 2003. Waterbirth and song. In *Midwifery Best Practice*, ed. S. Wickham. UK: Books for Midwives.

Kitzinger, S. 2005. *The Politics of Birth*. London: Elsevier.

Kuusela, P. et al. 1998. Warm tub bath during opening phase of labor. *Suomen Laakarilehti* 11: 1217–21.

Laurance, J. 2007. Waterbirth – provides the safest form of pain relief. *The Independent* 26 September.

Leboyer, F. 1975. *Birth Without Violence*. London: Mandarin.

Leitch, C. R. and J. J. Walker. 1998. The rise in Caesarean section rate: the same indications but a lower threshold. *British Journal of Obstetrics and Gynaecology* 105(6) June: 621–6.

Lenstrup, C. et al. 1987. Warm tub bath during delivery. *Acta Obstetricia et Gynecologica Scandinavica* 66: 709–12.

Lester, O. 2008. First breath. *Midwifery Matters* 117 Summer: 11.

Lichy, R. and E. Herzberg. 1993. *The Waterbirth Handbook*. Bath: Gateway.

Longridge, C. N. 1908. *A Manual for Midwives*. London: Churchill.

Lopriore, E., G. F. van Burk, F. J. Walther and A. J. de Beaufort. 2004. Correct use of the Apgar score for resuscitated and intubated babies. *MIDIRS* 14(4): 534–5.

Macarthur, C. et al. 1990. Epidural anaesthesia and long term backache after childbirth. *BMJ* 301(6742) 7 July: 9–12.

Macaulay, J. H., K. Bond and P. J. Steer. 1992. Epidural analgesia in labor and fetal hyperthermia. *Obstetrics and Gynecology* 80(4): 665–9.

Mackay, M. M. 2001. Use of water in labor and birth. *Clinical Obstetrics and Gynecology* 44(4) December: 733–49.

Maltau, M. J. 1979. Effects of betamethasone on plasma levels of estriol, cortisol and hcg in late pregnancy. *Acta Obstetricia et Gynecologica Scandinavica* 58(3): 235–8.

Mayer, K. 2004. Great to VBAC at home. *Midwifery Matters* 103 Winter: 7–8.

McCandlish, R. and M. Renfrew. 1993. Immersion in water during labour and/or birth. *Birth* 20(2): 79– 85.

McCandlish, R. et al. 1998. A randomised controlled trial of care of the perineum during second stage of normal labour. *RCOG British Journal of Obstetrics and Gynaecology* 105 December: 1262–72.

McCandlish, R. and L. A. Page. 2006. Being with Jane in childbirth: putting science and sensitivity into practice. In *New Midwifery: Science and Sensitivity in Practice* (2nd edn). Oxford: Churchill Livingstone.

McCraw, R. K. 1989. Recent innovations in childbirth. *Journal of Nursing Midwifery* 34(4): 206–10.

McDonald, S. 1999. Physiological and management of the third stage of labour. In V. R. Bennett and L. K. Brown (eds), *Myle's Textbook for Midwives* (15th edn). London: Churchill Livingstone.

Melzak, R. and P. D. Wall. 1965. Pain mechanism: a new theory. *Science* 150(3699): 971–9.

Mercer, J. S. 2001. Current best evidence: a review of the literature on umbilical cord clamping. *Journal of Midwifery and Women's Health* 46(6) November/ December: 402–14.

Miller, J. M. and J. Magill-Cuerden. 2006. All women in labour should have the choice of waterbirth. *British Journal of Midwifery* 14(8) August: 484–5.

Milner, I. 1988. Waterbabies. *Nursing Times* 84(1): 39–40.

Napierela, S. 1994. *Waterbirth: A Midwife's Perspective*. Westport, CN: Bergin and Garvey.

Newburgh, L. H. 1968. *Physiology of Heat Regulation and the Science of Clotting*. New York: Hafner.

Newburn, M. and D. Singh. 2003. *Creating a Better Birth Environment*. London: NCT.

NICE (National Institute for Clinical Excellence). 2004. *Caesarean Section*. London: NHS.

NICE (National Institute for Health and Clinical Excellence). 2007. *Intrapartum Care*. London: NHS.

Nicol, G. 1975. *Finland*. London: Batsford.

Nicoll. A., K. Hoggins and P. Winters. 2004. Waterbirth – changing attitudes. *AIMS Journal* 1(7).

Nightingale, C. 1994. Water birth in practice. *Modern Midwife* January: 15–19.

Nikoderm, C. et al. 1999. The effects of water on birth: a randomized controlled trial. 14th Conference on Priorities in Perinatal Care in South Africa. March, South Africa

Nikoderm, V. 2004. *Immersion in Water in Pregnancy, Labour and Birth*. Cochrane Review in Cochrane Library, Issue 1. Chichester: John Wiley.

NMC. 2004. *Midwives' Rules and Standards*. London: NMC.

NMC. 2006. *Standards for the Preparation and Practice of Supervisors of Midwives*. London: NMC.

Nyman, L. 1999. Waterbirth and the risk of infection. A case control study. ICM Conference Proceedings, Manila.

Ockenden, J. 2001. Water labour and birth. *The Practising Midwife* 4(9): 30–2.

Odent, M. 1981. The evolution of obstetrics in Pithiviers. *Birth and the Family* 8(1): 7–15.

Odent, M. 1983. Birth under water. *Lancet* December 24/31: 1476–7.

Odent, M. 1984. *Entering the World*. London: Marion Boyers.

Odent, M. 1987. The fetus ejection reflex. *Birth* 14(2): 104–5.

Odent, M. 1990. *Water and Sexuality*. London: Arkana.

Odent, M. 1998. *Entering the World*. London: Marion Boyers.

Ohlsson, G., P. Buchhave, U. Leandersson, L. Nordstrom, H. Rydhstrom and I. Sjolin. 2001. Warm tub bathing during labor: maternal and neonatal effects. *Acta Obstetricia et Gynecologica Scandinavica* 80: 311–14.

O'Sullivan, G., B. Liu, D. Hart et al. 2009. Effect of food intake during labour on obstetric outcome: randomized controlled trial. *BMJ* 338: b784.

Otigbah, C. M. et al. 2000. A retrospective comparison of water births and conventional vaginal deliveries. *European Journal of Obstetrics and Gynaecology and Reproductive Biology* 91: 15–20.

Page, L. A. and R. McCandlish. 2006. *The New Midwifery* (2nd edn). London: Churchill Livingstone.

Pairman, S. J. Pincombe and C. Thorogood. 2006. *Midwifery – Preparation for Practice*. Australia: Elsevier.

Palanisamy, A. et al. 2007. Fever, epidurals and inflammation: a burning issue. *Journal of Clinical Anaesthesia* 19(3) May.

Pearce, J. C. 1977. *Magical Child*. London: Paladin Granada.

Perlman, J. M. 2006. Hyperthermia in the delivery: potential impact on neonatal mortality and morbidity. *Clinics in Perinatology* 33(1) March: 55–63.

Pinette, M. G., J. Wax and E. Wilson. 2004. The risks of underwater birth. *American Journal of Obstetrics and Gynecology* 190: 1211–15.

Plumb, J., D. Holwell, R. Burton and P. Steer. 2007. Water birth for women with GBS: a pipe dream? *Practising Midwife* 10(11): 27–9.

Ponette, H. 1996. *Waterbirths*. New aquatic centre presentation. Aquarius.

Ponette, H. 1999. *Waterbirths in the 21st Century*. Aquarius.

Power, G. G. 1989. Biology of temperature: the mammalian fetus. *Journal of Developmental Physiology* 12: 295–304.

Ray, S. 1986. *Ideal Birth*. USA: Celestial Arts.

RCM. 1997. *Normality in Midwifery*. London: RCM.

RCM. 2006. *Masterly Inactivity. 2006 Campaign for Normal Birth*. London: RCM.

RCM, RCOG, NCT. 2007. *Making Normal Birth a Reality*. Consensus Statement from the Maternity Care Working Party. London: MCWP.

RCOG. 2003. *Clinical Green Top Guidelines. Prevention of Early Onset Neonatal Group B Streptococcal Disease*. London: RCOG.

RCOG. 2007. *Safer Childbirth: Minimum Standards for the Organization and Delivery of Care in Labour*. London: RCOG.

RCOG and RCM. 2006. *Immersion in Water during Labour and Birth*. London.

Redwood, R. 1999. Caring control: methodological issues in a discourse analysis of waterbirth texts. *Journal of Advanced Nursing* 2994: 914–21.

Reed, R. 2007. Nuchal cords: think before you check. *The Practising Midwife* 10(5) May: 18–20.

Reed, B. 2008. Sheelagh's story. *The Practising Midwife* 11(6) June: 28–31.

Reid-Campion, M. 1990. *Adult Hydrotherapy*. Oxford: Heinemann.

Richmond, H. 2003. Theories surrounding waterbirth. *The Practising Midwife* 6(2): 10–13.

Richmond, H. 2003. Women's experience of waterbirth. *The Practising Midwife* 6(3) March: 26–31.

Riggs, M. 1991. *The Scented Bath*. London: Robert Hale.

Robertson, A. 2002. Are midwives a dying breed? *The Practising Midwife* 5(7): 16.

Rosenthal, M. 1991. Warm water immersion in labor and birth. *The Female Patient* 16: 35.

Rosevear, S. et al. 1993. Birthing pools and the fetus. *Lancet* 342: 1048–9.

Royal Australian and New Zealand College of Obstetricians and Gynaecologists. 2008. *Warm Water Immersion during Labour and Birth*. Melbourne, Australia.

Rush, J. et al. 1996. The effects of whirlpool baths in labour: a randomized controlled trial. *Birth* 23(3): 136–43.

Sadan, O., S. E. Fleischfarb, A. Golan and S. Lurie. 2007. Cord around the neck: should it be severed at delivery? A randomized controlled study. *American Journal of Perinatology* 24(1) January: 61–4.

Schorn, M. et al. 1993. Water immersion and the effect on labor. *Journal of Nurse Midwifery* 6: 336–42.

Schroeter, K. 2004. Waterbirths – a naked emperor. *Paediatrics* September: 855–8.

Sellar, M. 2008. The VBAC waterbirth experience in Fife. *Midwives* August/September: 18–19.

Sidenbladh, E. 1983. *Waterbabies*. London: Adam and Charles Black.

Siegel, P. 1960. Does bath water enter the vagina? *Obstetrics and Gynaecology* 15: 660–1.

Simkin, P. 1986. Stress pain and catecholamines in labour. *Birth* 13(4) December: 227–33.

Simkin, P. 1990. Hydrotherapy. *Effective Care in Pregnancy and Childbirth* 2: 898–9.

Skinner, A. T. et al. 1986. *Duffield's Exercise in Water*. London: Bailliere Tindall.

Smirnov, I. V. 2002. The effect of water environment on the psychosomatic development of babies. *Explore* 11(6): 1–3.

Stables, D. and J. Rankin. 2005. *Physiology in Childbearing*. Oxford: Elsevier.

Stanway, A. 1979. *Alternative Medicine*. London: McDonalds and James.

Star, R. B. 1986. *The Healing Power of Birth*. Austin, TX: Star.

Stewart, M. 2001. Whose evidence counts? *Midwifery* 17: 279–88.

Stockton, A. 2009. Marly's birth story. *AIMS Journal* 21(4): 16–17.

Sumpter, Y. 2001. Waterbirth mother accused of illegal birth and child neglect. *AIMS Journal* 13(1) Spring: 7–9.

Taha, M. 2000. Water as a method of pain relief: a randomized controlled trial. 20th Conference on Priorities in Perinatal Care in Southern Africa.

Thni, A. and K. Mussner. 2003. Study shows benefits of underwater birth. *Geburtshilfe und Frauenheilkunde* 62: 977.

Thoeni, N., N. Zech, L. Moroder and F. Ploner. 2005. Review of 1600 water births. Does water birth increase the risk of neonatal infection? *Journal of Maternal, Fetal and Neonatal Medicine* 17(5) May: 357–61.

Tiran, D., and S. Mack. 2000. *Complementary Therapies for Pregnancy and Childbirth* (2nd edn). London: Balliere Tindall.

UKCC. 1994. *Position Statement on Waterbirths*. London: UKCC.

Verny, T. 1987. *The Secret Life of the Unborn Child*. London: Sphere.

Walsh, D. 2002. What is a 'normal midwife'? The research midwife's view. *The Practising Midwife* 5(7): 12–13.

Walsh, D. 2007. *Evidence-based Care for Normal Labour and Birth*. London: Routledge.

Walsh, D. 2009. Pain and epidural use in normal childbirth. Evidence-based practice. RCM Annual Event, Belfast.

Wambach, H. 1979. *Life before Life*. London: Bantam.

Wattis, L. J. 2001. The third stage maze – which practice pathway for optimal outcomes? *The Practising Midwife* 4(4): 23–7.

Weston, C. F. M. et al. 1987. Haemodynamic changes in man during immersion in water at different temperatures. *Clinical Science* 73: 613–16.

WHO. 1996. *Care in Normal Birth. A Practical Guide*. Geneva: WHO.

WHO. 1999. *Care of Normal Birth: A Practical Guide*. Report of the technical working group. Geneva: WHO.

Wickham, S. 1999. Further thoughts on the third stage. *The Practising Midwife* 2(10): 14–15.

Wickham, S. 2003. *Midwifery Best Practice*. Cheshire: BFM.

Wickham, S. 2006. *Midwifery Best Practice*. Butterworth Heinemann.

Widdecombe, J. 2004. Henry Head and his paradoxical reflex. *Journal of Physiology* 15(559) (part1) August: 1–2.

Wielder, I. 1999. *Inward Journey – Outward Bound*. Wielder, New Mexico.

Winterton Report. 1992. House of Commons Health Committee. Second Report – Maternity services. London: HMSO.

Woodward, J. 2004. A pilot study for a randomized controlled trial of waterbirth versus landbirth. *BJOG – International Journal of Obstetrics and Gynaecology* 111(6): 537–45.

Woodward, J. et al. 2004. A pilot for a RCT of waterbirth versus land birth. *MIDIRS* 14(3): 361–9.

Wu, C. J. and U. L. Chung. 2003. The decision making experience of mothers selecting waterbirth. *Journal of Nursing Research* 11(4): 261–8.

Wylie, L. 2005. *Essential Anatomy and Physiology in Maternity Care*. Oxford: Elsevier.

Yao, A. C. and J. Lind. 1974. Placental transfusion. *American Journal of Diseases of Children* 127: 128–41.

Yeates, D. A. et al. 1984. A comparison of two bearing down techniques during the second stage of labour. *Journal of Nurse Midwifery* 29: 3–11.

Zanetti-Dallenbach, R., O. Lapaire, A. Maertens, R. Frei, W. Holzgreve and I. Hosli. 2006. Waterbirth: is the water an additional reservoir for group B streptococcus? *Archives of Gynaecology and Obstetrics* 273: 236–8.

Zimmerman, R. 1993. Waterbirth – is it safe? *Journal of Perinatal Medicine* 21: 5–11.

Index